super

sexual

Orgasm

**Discover
the Ultimate
Pleasure Spot:
The Cul-de-sac**

Also by Barbara Keesling, Ph.D.

Talk Sexy to the One You Love
How to Make Love All Night
Sexual Healing
Sexual Pleasure: Reaching New Heights of Sexual Arousal
  and Intimacy

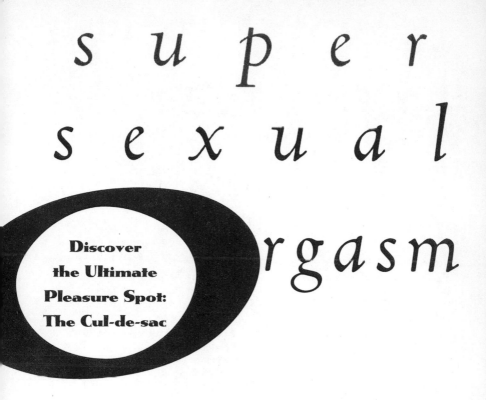

super sexual Orgasm

Discover the Ultimate Pleasure Spot: The Cul-de-sac

Barbara Keesling, Ph.D.

■ HarperCollins*Publishers*

Designed by Elina D. Nudelman

ISBN 0-06-017479-X

Contents

Introduction

Within every woman's body lies the potential for a vaginal orgasm so explosive and so consuming that, once experienced, it immediately and permanently redefines a woman's understanding of her own sexuality. This *super sexual orgasm*—an instantaneous vaginal orgasm triggered by penetration—is the ultimate sexual pleasure. This book is your guide to that pleasure. It is a road map to changing your life. And it is a gift I am very anxious to share with you.

As a sex therapist, nothing has been more important to me than understanding the phenomenon we call orgasm. And nothing is more exciting to me, both professionally and personally, than super sexual orgasm. Today, after almost twenty years of professional work in the field of human sexuality I feel confident in my ability to finally make this little known secret *every* woman's secret. Today, *every* woman can experience super sexual orgasm, and in the pages that follow I am going to teach you everything you need to know to open the door to your first super sexual orgasm, or SSO. The exercises and the techniques, the positions to make it easier—even instructions and support for your partner—they're all here.

On the lighter side, I have been called the "Martha Stewart of Sex" and "the first sex therapist who looks like she's had sex." On a more serious note, I am a sex therapist in California, with a private practice at the Riskin-Banker Psychotherapy Center in Santa Ana. I received my Ph.D. in Health Psychology and have been teaching courses at California colleges on human sexuality and psychopathology for many years.

Prior to becoming a therapist I was a professional sex surrogate. When an individual comes to a sex therapist for problems such as lack of desire or orgasm, many sex therapists work with professional surrogate partners who act as the client's partner during therapy. Some of my greatest insights into human sexuality have been derived from my twelve years of working as a surrogate partner, including many of my insights into super sexual orgasm.

I believe sex is one of the purest forms of human endeavor. Sex is kaleidoscopic in its expressive and experiential possibility. It can be joyously exuberant. It can be a thrilling adventure into the unknown. It can be soothing and centering. Sex cuts to the core of who you are as an individual. It is the ultimate arena of sharing between people. It is the nourishing confluence of so many special elements: touch, physicality, communication, play, genital activity, arousal, orgasm, and intimacy. I also believe sex has an unparalleled power to heal us and our partners on an emotional, physical, and spiritual level.

Of all the things I have learned in my journeys as a woman, a sex therapist, a healer, a teacher, and a partner, super sexual orgasm stands alone. To me, super sexual orgasm is the sexual holy grail, the centerpiece for body, mind, and spirit integration for every woman. The relevance for women is universal.

One of the most beautiful and unique aspects of the SSO experience is that it provides what most women yearn for in their intimate lives: control. This one word is *pivotal* to female sexuality.

Women want to have control when they make love. When I say women want to have control, I'm not talking about women wanting to be dominatrices or women wanting to be on top—which is what you might think I am talking about. I'm saying this: Women want to have control of their sexual energies. They want to fully enjoy every scintilla of their lovemaking, from sensual caressing to supersonic climaxes. They want to take advantage of every possibility for pleasure. Doesn't this ring true for you?

Super sexual orgasm will put you in control. The preparation will awaken you to your sexual energies, rhythms, and strength. And once you discover the magic of SSO, you will be able to decide if you want to have your explosive climax at the beginning of intercourse *or* wait till your partner is on the verge of orgasm *or* have multiple explosive orgasms *or* have it all! All of this will be available to you. You will have the control. Isn't this what you want?

There is a line of thought that maintains that to be fully womanly means surrendering to male sexual prowess and power during lovemaking. I'm not sure where that attitude started but I find many of my female therapeutic clients and many of the women who attend my lectures or speak at my talk show appearances sincerely adhere to that view . . . until they understand and access their own personal SSO experience.

When you are in control with the extraordinary power of super sexual orgasm—able to mobilize your sexual and sensual essence and exercise it when you want it and how you want it—you do in fact surrender. But you know in every fiber of your body that you are surrendering not to the supremacy of your partner, but to your own volatile, deliciously consuming sexuality.

Now, this is not to say that making super sexual orgasm your own means you are facing the world like a Mack truck! What SSO will do for you is much more subtle. It allows you to find and become the essential in you. It gives you confidence, it gives you strength, and it gives you the keys to your own pleasure.

For many women, having orgasms has become a point of pressure, disappointment, and even unhappiness. This needs to change. My intention is to free women to enjoy their orgasms and simultaneously take the pressure off having orgasms. But to get there, we need to start from a very different place. We need to start by accessing and understanding your full sexual potential as a woman and your full orgasmic capacity. When you are in command of your own body, understand its vast sexual potential and can access this potential at your choosing, then performance anxieties dissolve, and you can revel in what your body has to offer. Learn all there is to learn, feel all there is to feel; then you are truly free.

Super sexual orgasm is a comprehensive experience. It

doesn't just feel fabulous, it changes lives. It gives you control. It lets you surrender. And it overwhelms you with pleasure. But if you are going to welcome SSO into your life, you will need to prepare on many levels:

- SSO requires a level of muscular strength and coordination that you have probably never needed before to experience erotic pleasure. This means taking a little time to build up areas in the body you have probably given little notice to before.

- SSO requires that you are more comfortable with your body than you have probably ever been before—*all* of your body, including the most intimate areas.

- SSO requires that you are more comfortable with your partner than you may have ever been before. You are going to need your partner's help and support, and you are going to need to feel a clear bond of trust.

To make all of this possible for you, and to keep the process a simple one, I have divided this book into two sections. In Part I we will focus on the exercises and techniques that will bring your body to a state of readiness, and you will experience your first super sexual orgasm. Part II will focus on integrating SSO into your emotional life, with special emphasis on strengthening the bonds of your partnership. As with so many other aspects of female sexuality and erotic pleasure, there is much more involved in SSO than a mechanical "now do this, then do that" approach. We need to address the issues of comfort and trust, and we need to address the space of permission you must be in to fully experience SSO.

By the time you have completed both sections, body, mind, and spirit will have all been well attended to, and super sexual orgasm will be yours to enjoy for the rest of your life.

From my contact with thousands of women worldwide I know that women are ready to embrace their true and full sexual potential. I know they are ready for the most profound sensual experience of their lives. I know you are, and I promise that super sexual orgasm will bring much joy and love into your life. You do not have to long for it. You can claim it right now. And all you have to do is turn the page.

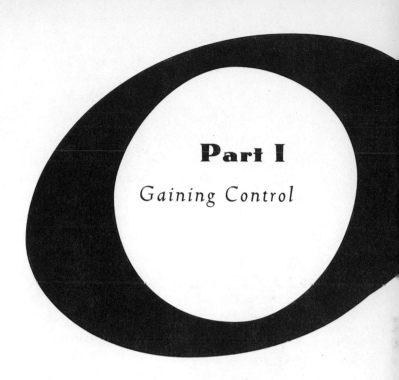

Part I

Gaining Control

1

Secrets

You are about to experience an orgasm that is going to shatter every notion you have ever had about the joys of making love. Whether you are a highly orgasmic woman who regularly enjoys deep sensual fulfillment or you are one of the silent majority of women who has to work hard to achieve a satisfying erotic connection, your understanding of your own orgasmic potential is about to change forever.

Imagine, if you will, an explosive vaginal orgasm that doesn't require prolonged intercourse to the point of exhaustion. Imagine an explosive vaginal orgasm that

does not require convoluted gymnastics or a perfect partner. Imagine an explosive vaginal orgasm that never dis-
appoints you and never fails. Imagine an explosive vaginal
orgasm that *you* control. That's a super sexual orgasm.

PAM'S SECRET

I am a sex therapist in private practice in Southern
California, but I actually began my work in the field of
human sexuality as a sexual surrogate. When I first
started my work years ago as a surrogate partner, there
was another surrogate working at the same clinic—let's
call her Pam—who was able to have, according to her,
the most deliciously powerful vaginal orgasms, instanta-
neously triggered at penetration. Pam had always had
these "vaginal volcanoes" as she described them to me.
She said the experience was all-consuming and enor-
mously, deliciously spellbinding. Her orgasms had never
been any different and she actually thought hers was
every woman's experience!

It was so tantalizingly frustrating for me to hear how
Pam could offer no explanation for how others could
replicate her enormous pleasure. It also seemed strange
from a research perspective that such an enormous
potential for a woman's pleasure was so little understood.
After all, I thought, if we can put satellites in the sky that
can read the license plate of the car in your driveway,
surely we can figure out Pam's secret!

Well, it wasn't always easy but I was very determined.
Over the years, my therapeutic work and the work of my

colleagues moved me closer and closer to discovering Pam's secret. And finally, after many years, all of the pieces of the puzzle came together. Finally, I was able to understand what Pam's body had been doing. And, even more important, Pam's secret became a secret that could be shared.

INTRODUCING THE KEY TO PLEASURE: THE CUL-DE-SAC

The key to super sexual orgasm lies within a small passage of the vaginal canal, just beyond the cervix, known as the cul-de-sac. As is so often the case with labels, the name of this passage belies the truth, for this cul-de-sac is no dead end. To the contrary, this small section of the vaginal canal is so extraordinarily rich in sensitive nerve endings that the slightest contact with a man's penis or sex toy can trigger an instantaneous orgasm so powerful, so shiveringly all-consuming, and so absolutely delicious that it practically defies description (though the phrase "lightning bolt" does come to mind!).

This cul-de-sac passage is the gateway to total erotic pleasure. And the "cul-de-sac response" that is triggered during penetration is the secret that is about to change your life. Sounds simple, doesn't it? It is simple. Beautifully simple. But here's the problem: While every woman has a cul-de-sac, not every woman can make this super-charged part of the vaginal canal "available" during intercourse. For most women, the weight and positioning of the uterus tend to compress the vaginal canal at the entrance to the cul-de-sac passage, creating a daunting vaginal roadblock. This most unwelcome obstruction tends to make the special cul-de-sac passage a closed road, inaccessible to penetration by the penis during intercourse. The penis (or dildo) may reach, but it cannot enter, and as a result, the most potentially gratifying erotic experience any woman could imagine remains just out of reach. Out of reach, that is, until now.

Over the past several years I have worked with my colleagues and clients to develop a simple program of exercises and techniques to give a woman the necessary strength and control in her uterus and vagina to actually lift and flatten the uterus during intercourse, to "fan" the vaginal canal, and open the cul-de-sac passage to penetration. The result: super sexual orgasm in the cul-de-sac passage for any woman who has the desire to make it possible.

This program is included in its entirety in Part I. It begins with exercises to build necessary muscle strength and control (Chapter 2). It continues with exercises and techniques to help you capture necessary body motion and positioning (Chapter 3). And it culminates in a powerful synthesis that will bring you to your first super sexual orgasm (Chapter 4).

SUPER SEXUAL ORGASM IS A CHALLENGE EASILY MET

The program I have just described may sound complicated or daunting. It may even sound absolutely exhausting. But it isn't. The entire program can be completed in less than a few weeks, practicing only *minutes* per day. Minutes! It's fast, it's fun, it's sexy, and it's foolproof. It all feels fabulous, and it's truly *easy*. Best of all, it will give you the potential for a *lifetime* of pleasure.

And if it all sounds a little too good to be true, you should know that there are a substantial number of women who have already experienced super sexual orgasm. While some of these women are clients who have learned the secret of the cul-de-sac from me or one of my fellow clinicians, most are not. Like Pam, whose story I've already told you, these are just very lucky women—lucky because their uterus lifts and flattens naturally and automatically when they are sufficiently aroused during intercourse, and the exquisitely sensitive cul-de-sac becomes open to penetration.

While the majority of these women may not know the exact details of what is happening within their vaginal canal to make their orgasms so powerful, what all of these women *do* know is the explosion of sensation that is triggered by intimate contact with their partner's penis in this very special passage.

Many of these women actually believe that their orgasms are perfectly normal. After all, it's normal for them. And these same women are almost always surprised to learn that other women don't experience half of the orgasm that they can experience *regularly* during intercourse. But the fact is that the vast majority of women are nowhere near as lucky as this relatively small group of "natural" success stories. The fact is that the vast majority of women could have intercourse for an entire lifetime without ever experiencing any of these exquisite sensations. But that doesn't mean they have to.

Today, *every* woman can experience super sexual orgasm, and I am going to show you how. But first, I want to talk to you about arousal and orgasm.

MORE SECRETS

Maybe you already know everything there is to know about the physiology of arousal and orgasm. But my clinical practice has shown me that many women are positively mystified by both processes. Some of the explanations I've heard are so wacky I'd swear I was hearing excerpts from a stand-up comedy routine.

You see, we take our birth control pills, have our diaphragms or condoms at the ready. We have our copies of *Our Bodies, Our Selves* hanging around the house somewhere in case we need to look up something in an emergency. We think we are pretty much sexually self-responsible. But how much do we really know? It's like the people in the old days who considered themselves to be well-informed when they thought the world was flat: There was a gap between reality and their understanding of it. And there is a similar gap between the reality of what it takes to be sexually well-informed and many women's understanding of their bodies.

Now fortunately, we have the information about what happens during arousal and orgasm. The issue isn't lack of details on this matter. The issue is that most women have seen no reason to obtain this knowledge. Somehow we get aroused, have an orgasm, and that's that. As for the rest of what's involved? Whatever.

No more "whatever." The motivation for knowing is here. In order to work toward increasing your orgasmic ability to an SSO level, you need to have a complete understanding of your sexual functioning. During your SSO you are of course not going to be saying, Now there goes this and there goes that. But to get to that point of total release and abandon where you are not paying attention you have to pay attention in the beginning—starting now.

Aroused and Aware

When you become physically sexually aroused, blood moves from the periphery of your body to the center, especially to the genital area. The vulva and clitoris enlarge and sometimes become a deeper red or pink. Usually you become lubricated: Fluid is produced inside the vagina and along the inner lips by the increased blood flow in this area, causing the tissue walls to "sweat." You may have noticed you have little to no lubrication. Do not be alarmed. Some women just don't and instead rely on oils from baby oil to KY jelly. (Remember, if you have a minimal lubrication reflex do not let your partner stimulate you until you apply oil, otherwise you will find yourself experiencing pain and irritation.)

You can try to stimulate and increase your lubrication reflex—the glands called the Bartholin's glands—by slowly caressing your clitoris, inner and outer lips, and perineum. Gently rest your fingers alongside the sides of the vaginal opening halfway between your clitoris and perineum. Steady but light touching of this area will help stimulate the Bartholin's glands.

In addition to arousal in the genitals, your body's experience of arousal can include faster, deeper breathing, increased heart rate, and a psychological feeling of pleasure. Note, however, something you may have experienced yourself from time to time: You can be aroused physically but not psychologically. The body's experience is only half of the equation, and this is something that both women and men need to be fully cognizant of. Otherwise, there is great room for misunderstanding and confusion.

Reaching the Climax

There are a number of ways in which women have orgasms. Stimulation of the clitoris, for instance, can produce orgasm. Some women can also have one from fondling their breasts, especially the nipples. Other areas that can trigger orgasm include the cervix; the opening of the urethra; the G-spot, located on the upper wall of the vagina; the cul-de-sac (soon to be your new best friend); and the pubococcygeous (PC) muscle (much more on this area in particular in our next chapter). Some women experience orgasm with no physical stimulation at all. They can wake from an erotic dream and have one.

Before continuing with this discussion about climax,

let's take a quick look at the physiology of intercourse. During penetration, your PC muscle will tighten around the penis, vibrator, or dildo, and the vaginal walls will tighten as well. Penetration can also cause rubbing up against the G-spot, cervix (which some women find pleasant while others do not), the cul-de-sac (if the uterus flattens and lifts), and the ovaries. If this last possibility occurs, especially during ovulation, you may experience great discomfort, even pain. During penetration, the vaginal walls may be caressed. They contain striations or "rugae" that when rubbed can actually be felt as bumps by both women and men. In addition, parts of the vagina may balloon out or tighten during intercourse.

Despite the existence of so many body areas in which orgasms can be triggered, many women have never experienced a single climax. Still others remain confused about what is actually taking place. Every woman, of course, experiences her orgasm in an idiosyncratic way, but generally having an orgasm goes like this: The muscles around your uterus and cervix spasm so that your abdomen sucks in or flutters. You may expel some air from your vagina. Your blood pressure, heart rate, and breathing all reach a peak. Your neck, arms, and legs may spasm involuntarily and moments later so does your PC muscle. You may feel a tingling sensation in some parts of your body and a warmth that moves from your genitals up to your chest, neck, and face. All the energy created in this process is then rapidly discharged as you feel physically and psychologically released. For the same woman orgasms can vary in intensity. Some may include only PC muscle spasms and a mild, good feeling. Others may be so strong they cause your body to arch off the bed.

I am going over all of this with you because I want you to be confident and comfortable in the knowledge that all orgasms, regardless of magnitude, occur in the same way for every woman. This includes super sexual orgasms. It is not a question of some women being better at orgasms than others. Your body gives you what it has and whatever it is should be appreciated as a beautiful, loving experience. What is important, and why you are reading this book, is to open yourself completely to your maximum orgasmic capacity and delight in it to the hilt.

A COMPREHENSIVE PROGRAM, A GUARANTEED SUCCESS

In the chapters that follow I will slowly and methodically lay out all of the exercises and techniques you will need to completely prepare yourself to welcome SSO into your life. These exercises attend to every critical muscle, every critical movement, and every critical feeling, and they are presented in an order that maximizes their impact—an order I would ask you to follow. I hope I've anticipated all the questions you might have for me along the way and done my best to answer them. As always, though, if you are left with any questions or concerns, you can write to me in care of my publisher.

At times, a given exercise or group of exercises may seem superfluous, repetitive, off-track, or even silly. You need to know that every single exercise in this program has been included for a very specific reason. I want to be absolutely certain that each and every woman who picks up this book will have the consummate experience she is looking for. And to ensure this, I have left no stone unturned. I promise you that by the time you have completed the program it will all make perfect sense, and you will have what you are hoping for: the perfect super sexual orgasm.

Some of the techniques we will be exploring in the book are preparatory, that is to say, more like a training to condition your body physically to engage in the SSO process. Other techniques will actually be those you use during the lovemaking experience. As you become familiar with these techniques they will become second nature to you and feel less like a structure. Think of these techniques as a sugar cube on your tongue. At the beginning, in order to get the sweetness you have to have the sensation of a cube dissolving into you. Then you experience the sweetness as a part of yourself.

This is not mission impossible, nor is it mission forever. You are guaranteed to make progress if you work consistently, thoroughly, and honestly. In terms of time, we're talking about a range of three weeks on average, depending on your own body response and rhythms.

For some women, this may still sound like a lot, maybe even a bit too much. That's okay. If you need to streamline things, use your judgment to decide which aspects are most crucial for your development right now. Modify exercises, if you wish, to suit your needs. And, if necessary, eliminate those you feel you have already attended to satisfactorily at another time. If you are a regular and devout practitioner of Kegel exercises, for example, don't feel the need to augment your program here.

Use your good sense and it is not likely you will make a mistake. But always know that following the program page by page, in its absolute entirety, is your guaranteed road to SSO success.

A WORD TO THE WISE

It is very important that you understand right here and now that this is not a book about just a few square inches of space deep within the vagina. Nor is it a typical "plumbing manual" or a blueprint for a clinical exploration. Indeed, I would be doing you a great disservice to focus exclusively on the cul-de-sac passage. It would be no different than embracing the insensitive attitudes of years ago that viewed female sexuality as beginning and ending in the vagina.

Yes, super sexual orgasm does indeed come to fruition in the cul-de-sac passage, where it is triggered. But there is more to SSO than the mere stimulation of the cul-de-sac passage. The cul-de-sac passage does not stand alone and apart. And super sexual orgasm begins not just in the body, but in the mind and in the spirit as well. The experience is comprehensive, and the preparation is comprehensive, but it is not difficult. None of this is difficult. But it does require a commitment to trusting my expertise and following my entire plan.

SHARE IT WITH YOUR PARTNER, SHARE IT WITH YOUR FRIENDS

The information I am writing about in this book on super sexual orgasm is intended for use by all women, whether in a monogamous sexual relationship or not. I even hope that some men will read it to expand their empathic sexual horizons. Let me make it clear at the outset, however, that a discussion of the "rightness" or "wrongness" of sex without commitment will not enter into these pages.

For some, sex whenever and with whomever is the essence of being alive. For others, it is essential to have such intimate contacts within the boundaries of a committed relationship. Personally, I believe in commitment and I believe in monogamy. But I do not believe in judging anyone else's needs or practices.

To put it very simply, sex is my life. As a sex therapist I have dedicated my career to helping others maximize their sensual enjoyment in positive, humanistic ways. But this necessitates leaving all judgments behind. Believe me when I tell you that I know all about sexual judgments. While I was fortunate to grow up in relaxed, sunny Southern California, I also grew up in a restrictive religious family. Once I tapped into the wealth of joy and excitement that good, healthy sex can bring I never looked back and never had any misgivings about the path I chose to tread. But above all, I left all judgments behind. As long as I can bring to my clients, readers like you, and lecture audiences around the world new insights into lovemaking I will feel that each day of my life was a day well spent.

So please embrace the openness within you and use it to facilitate your path to pleasure. I promise you that irrespective of the nature of your relationship or relationships, having super sexual orgasms will be a life-changing experience.

BEFORE YOU GET STARTED

You're probably anxious to get started, and it won't be long now—the program begins shortly with the first group of exercises you will find in Chapter 2. But one last word of caution: Once you begin the exercise program, *please do not look for any big shortcuts to the SSO payoff.*

I have been teaching SSO techniques to women for many years, and I know that it takes a thorough, multi-faceted approach—a mind, body, spirit approach—to reach the worthwhile goal of super sexual orgasm. Big shortcuts rarely work, and almost never work well, and this goes double for SSO. All of your channels need to be open. The physical channel (i.e., the cul-de-sac passage) most importantly, but also the emotional and spiritual channels that make up who you are as a woman. I have attended to all of this in this book. Please value my experience.

SSO transcends. And it is worth every drop of work to get there. This is not to say that the program is hard. I can say with complete confidence that it is never hard. But, as I have already said, it *is* comprehensive. So take your time. Proceed at your own pace. Treat every new discovery with the reverence it deserves. And enjoy every gorgeous moment along the way, because there is so much to enjoy. Yet always know that when you finally do arrive at your destination, indescribable magic will be there to greet you.

As you begin your journey toward extreme sexual pleasure and a profound understanding of yourself, please:

- be kind to you

- treat the exercise process we will be exploring with respect and not as a 100-meter dash—you are learning for a lifetime, not just for your next sexual encounter

- take the time to let the feeling of the exercises sink into your body and become comfortable to you

- remember to breathe fully and deeply—some clients have gotten so intense about the process that they forget to take the slow, deep, richly air-circulating breaths that are so nourishing to the body and enhancing to our sexuality

- most of all, enjoy and have fun!

MY SINCEREST WISHES FOR YOU ON YOUR JOURNEY

The turning point in the history of women's sexuality is here, and it has a name: super sexual orgasm. This new reality begins right now. Women who have disappointing orgasms are women who are choosing to accept these orgasms. If you have the will, I have the way. The ultimate sexual power is within you, and it is time to unearth the buried treasure locked inside your body and embrace a new life!

Soon you will see—see and *feel*—how SSO connects you to your deepest female self. You are entitled to live sexually to your fullest and love sexually to the highest of orgasmic heights. May you emerge from the learning path of this book as the sexual, loving woman you know you have always been. Because *you are*. My encouragement and entire support are there for you as you make this journey your own.

2
Muscle

it's time to get to work. Right now, the greatest obstacle standing between any woman and extraordinary super sexual orgasm pleasure is a series of surprisingly simple muscle exercises. Muscles make sex happen. And certain muscles make sex a total happening. I'm not trying to be flip here and I'm not exaggerating at all. Muscles open doors of sensuality and feeling, and when it comes to SSO, muscles are crucial. So right now it is time to get those doors open so that the ultimate pleasure can be welcomed into your life.

Your SSO training will begin with a pleasurable breathing exercise to relax you and a sensual caressing technique to get you ready for all that is to come. Next comes a simple but crucial muscle lesson. From muscle theory, we'll move quickly to muscle fact with some hands-on practice. First, I'll teach you a gentle Kegel (PC muscle) exercise that many women are already familiar with, and we'll slowly build from there. As you get stronger, we'll be adding interesting ingredients into the mix. You'll have a chance to do sensuous strengthening exercises with a dildo, and I'm even going to ask you to give your G-spot a workout. Do you know what a "gusher" is? You will soon, and you will be so glad you do. Every exercise is here for a reason. None of this training is superfluous (it is, of course, all *fabulous*). All of it is in the service of your ultimate goal: super sexual orgasm. Breathing exercises, Kegel exercises, G-spot exercises, uterine exercises, vaginal muscle exercises, stomach exercises (even the caressing techniques) . . . they are all an important part of your SSO preparation.

DON'T GET OVERWHELMED, AND DON'T RUSH . . .

This is a very important chapter. And there is a lot in here. Please take it very, very slowly, letting yourself enjoy everything the way it was meant to be enjoyed. And please don't panic at the thought of a chapter of exercises involving parts of your body you were oblivious to before this moment. There is nothing to be scared of. This is not going to be sex therapy à la Camp Pendleton, with instructions like "Get on your back and give me one hundred Kegels!" I'm not a drill sergeant and I'm not a fitness fanatic. I'm a sex therapist who wants to share something wonderful with women who deserve something wonderful.

I also promise you this will not be icky, strange, or weird, like a bad biology experiment where you aim a flashlight, put your hand "down there," and push and pull at yourself. All these exercises are medically sound, clinically proven, safe, and designed to be done with the utmost discretion and privacy.

If doing exercises makes you groan you'll be delighted to discover that my exercises make you moan . . . and smile . . . and feel sexy and in control of the most intimate parts of your body. Remember also to bring to the process the essential ingredients only you can give to yourself: gentleness, patience, and self-trust. *Allow what happens to happen.* Do not force anything on yourself. You are doing the best work you can do by exploring your natural self in a straightforward way.

I cannot predict exactly the nature of the sensations and journey you will have as you undertake the exercises in this chapter because your experience will be unique to you. I can tell you though that you will feel emotionally and physically many new and surprising, even startling, things as you explore the intimate workings of your body. Relax and enjoy these feel-good exercises, designed to empower your sexuality and your personal feminine strengths and to give you control over your own body.

Often times women at my lectures and workshops

have told me how these muscle exercises lifted an uneasiness that had been lingering in the back of their mind for many years—an uneasiness prompted by feelings they were strangers to their physical selves, especially their sexual-genital aspects. That's why I like to call these exercises "wholesome," because they are pure, natural, and feminine and because they give each woman who does them a sense of becoming profoundly whole.

It's your turn to experience this wonderful wholeness. Good for you for taking the steps to make this happen. Now, let's get started.

EVERY BREATH YOU TAKE

First, you need to learn how to "belly breathe." You will use this special breathing technique many times in your SSO training. You can also use belly breathing to relax before a sexual encounter, to relax you after a hard day's work, or to ground yourself whenever you need to feel more centered and calm.

Lie comfortably on your back. Place one hand on your abdomen. Slowly breathe in through your mouth. Breathe as if you are drawing breath down through your body, into your legs and toes. Then slowly exhale. Your stomach should rise and fall with this breath. Feel the air flowing all the way into your lungs and all the way out again. Visualize the air as a white light that relaxes and energizes at the same time. Do two or three belly breaths and then breathe normally for a couple of minutes. Do the belly breathing again. While doing this second round, *pause for three seconds between breathing out and breathing in. Don't pause between breathing in and breathing out. The inhale and exhale should be one seamless process. Do several more rounds of belly breathing in this manner. Breathe normally for a couple of minutes and then repeat the belly breathing cycle.*

THE SENSATE FOCUS CARESS

Sensate focus techniques are sensuous touching exercises designed to help men and women focus on, appreciate, and control the moment-to-moment experiences of contact, arousal, and release. Sensate focus techniques are not sex acts, and they are not masturbation techniques. They are very pleasurable ways of making contact with yourself or with a partner.

While there are many different sensate focus techniques, the only ones you need to learn for the purposes of this book are the full-body caress and the genital caress. Right now you are going to learn these by yourself. Later in the book, you will also practice with a partner. As you are practicing, remember that orgasm is not a goal of this exercise. Your only goal is to fully enjoy the pleasure of the sensations.

You will need a quiet room, preferably one that is free of distractions like ringing telephones. You will also need a lubricant such as baby oil, massage oil, cream, or KY jelly. KY jelly is usually the safest choice because it doesn't irritate the genitals. Be especially careful to have clean hands, and keep a clean towel handy.

Sit or lie naked on a comfortable surface or chair. Close your eyes and let yourself relax, using a belly breath to assist you.

The full-body caress begins by placing your fingertips on your body gently and focusing in on that point of contact. *Slowly explore the surface of your body with your fingertips, always maintaining contact with some part of your body.* Follow the point of contact wherever it moves—to your face, neck, shoulders, arms, etc.—and focus on what you are physically feeling at this contact point. If your mind wanders off into a sexual fantasy or into daily realities like errands or checkbook balancing, gently bring your mind back to the sensation being created by your touch.

Being touched in this manner is comforting and relaxing, which is necessary if you are to reach profound levels of arousal and SSO. Don't massage, but rather keep to a light, constant motion. You can use long sweeping strokes or short ones—try both styles to see what they do for you. You can use some type of lubrication if you like (I love scented oils!), but remember to warm them up in your hand before you apply them and maintain contact while you reapply them. Touch whatever you want in whatever order you want, but make sure to touch yourself all over. Breathe evenly and keep your eyes closed.

As you touch, let your sensory awareness include temperature, texture, shape, movement. If you find you are getting mechanical with your touch or getting bored, slow down. Chances are you aren't letting yourself really be in the moment. Try cutting your pace—even if you think it is superslow already—in half. Remember always that your only goal here is *to make yourself feel good.* Continue this for at least ten or fifteen minutes.

The genital caress begins when you are ready to shift the focus of your attention and touch to your genital area. This is not an occasion for masturbation. Right now you just need to caress slowly so that you can learn what kind of touch feels best, and where it feels best. Be especially careful to have clean hands and add a touch of baby oil or other lubricant before you proceed.

You may want to start by touching your breasts, stomach, or thighs, since they are all probably quite sensitive. Then slowly move to your inner thighs and outer vaginal lips. Keep your focus on what you are touching. Relax. Breathe. Next, slowly stroke your clitoris and the inner lips of your vagina. Feel their warmth and texture. Insert a finger into your vagina. Feel the warmth and texture of your vaginal walls. Let yourself explore and stay focused on the sensations. If you do become aroused, that's fine, but this is not the goal right now. Don't try not to make it happen, just allow what happens to happen.

If your mind drifts, remember to gently bring your focus back to the caress. Caress slowly. After twenty or thirty minutes, you can end the exercise, but feel free to continue longer.

MY FAVORITE MUSCLE

It's time to talk about muscles, and when I talk about muscles, I always like to start with a very small one that nevertheless deserves a very big introduction. Ladies, may I introduce the PC muscle! Believe me, I'm not overstating my case when I say the new era of sexual ful-fillment for women has arrived, heralded by the orgasmic potential of this one very special muscle. It is the muscle that defines orgasm, and it is the pivotal muscle in the cul-de-sac response.

While I know that some of you are already aware of the existence of the PC muscle, I also know that for the majority of you this is new territory. If you are reading about the PC here for the first time, know that this is perfectly okay. There is certainly no reason for you to feel out of the loop or out of touch with your body. It won't take long to get acquainted. And I give you my word, the initials PC are going to be emblazoned into your consciousness along with your shoe size after you have finished reading and performing the exercises in this chapter. You will never mistake PC for "politically correct." When you hear this term you will practically shiver as you associate it with the sublime ecstasy the PC muscle creates.

PC MUSCLE BASICS

The pubococcygeal muscle group (PC for short) is the first gatekeeper to your ultimate SSO pleasure, being directly tied in to cul-de-sac orgasm. The PC muscle group runs from the pelvic bone in the front of your body to your tailbone in the rear. This muscle group supports the floor of your pelvic cavity and your pelvic organs.

We will be working out with the PC muscle with an eye to increasing the heights of pleasure. Before we continue down this avenue, let me take a moment to mention that a toned PC muscle has other benefits for women as well: a better childbirth experience, quicker return of muscle tone after childbirth, and prevention and cure of incontinence.

The PC muscle actually first came to medical attention when physicians were working to correct bladder problems encountered by pregnant women. You may have heard of the word "Kegel." Some of the PC exercises that follow are referred to as Kegels because of their development by obstetrician Dr. A. H. Kegel.

In women, the PC muscle spasms during orgasm and gives the vagina a feeling of tightness. Men have a PC muscle too, by the way, which spasms when ejaculation occurs. Toning the PC muscle on a daily basis makes arousal, penetration, and orgasm more sexually intense because such strengthening tightens your vagina and builds muscle mass. The greater the mass, the more blood can collect in that area. This larger flow adds to the sensations during arousal and creates a greater sense of release when the PC muscle spasms during orgasm as the blood rushes back out. And just stimulating the PC muscle can produce orgasm—something you'll experience for yourself later.

Toning the PC muscle also overcomes a difficulty many women have: that of having an orgasm when there is a penis or some other object in their vagina. The PC muscle has to be quite strong to spasm fully during penetration. This is what the exercises are designed to address.

Locate your PC muscle by placing one of your fingers about one inch—up to the first knuckle—into the vagina. Internally, you should feel a drawing together or a drawing upward in your vaginal and pelvic area.

Squeeze as if you were stopping the flow of urination. The muscle that tightens around your finger as you do this is the PC muscle. That's it! Don't move another muscle. Don't confuse things by squeezing your tummy or your buttocks or your thighs. Just feel this one muscle. It may not feel very strong at this point; it may barely feel like a muscle. But this is the one and it's the one that counts.

If you are having trouble isolating this muscle, try consciously relaxing any surrounding muscles that may be confusing the picture for you. In other words, purposefully relax your stomach muscles. Purposefully relax your thighs and your buttocks. Now, once again, squeeze the muscle that you would squeeze to stop the flow of urination. Do you feel it more clearly now? Good.

I want you to squeeze again but before you do, check to see your breathing is not short and choppy from any anxiety you may have from doing this exercise. Because this exercise is connected with the sensual process of feminine excitement and orgasm you may need to take a few extra moments to relax right now. Belly breathe if you like. When you have settled and are breathing easily again, continue with the PC exercise. Flex the PC muscle again and make sure to keep your stomach, buttocks, thigh, and abdominal muscles relaxed as you do so. There, you did it!

Now that you know where the PC muscle is and what tightening it feels like, I want you to flex and relax the PC without using your finger to help. When you flex, hold it for two seconds before you release. Continue to breathe slowly and evenly the whole time, and use the belly breath if you need it. (If you are still having difficulty isolating the PC muscle from other pelvic muscles continue to use your finger as an aid; or perhaps you will find that flexing it to stop a flow of urination helps you determine what the action of the muscle feels like.)

Do a pattern of flexes, holds, and releases three times a day. In your first week, do six flexes in each set, the second week do twelve flexes in each set, and the third week do twenty flexes in each set. At this three-week point you'll have the firmness of muscle you need to achieve an SSO, when utilized in conjunction with the other techniques that follow in this and later chapters of the book.

After your initial training, I encourage you to continue doing these flexes every day (three times a day would be best), not only for the sake of your sex life and SSO but for your entire spectrum of health and well-being. The great thing about these flexes is that you can do them in the shower, on the bus, in the car, while you are watching television, just about any time. They can make even a boring mandatory company seminar or an endless home-owner's association meeting have a hidden appeal.

There is another huge payoff for dutifully performing your PC crunches: When used in combination with the other techniques you will learn in this chapter you will have the ability to literally grip objects that are inserted into your vagina—including your lover's penis! This will be a fantastic source of sexual pleasure not only for yourself but, as you can imagine, for your partner as well. Talk about motivation!

Now for those type-A personalities out there looking to be the speed-demons of sexuality, do not turn this into the Kegel 500 and do more than a few minutes of flexing three times a day. All you'll do is give yourself PC burnout. After all, the PC is a muscle and as with any muscle, if you overuse it, you'll feel tired and sore in that area. For those women who have had children, are over fifty, or who have not pared down to their desired weight yet, consider taking an extra week or weeks if necessary to build up to twenty flex repetitions.

Be attuned to what is going on with you. Don't just read what I write and apply it blindly. There is room for give and take in everything I'm describing in these chapters. Give yourself the time and attention you need to adjust all the exercises in this book to a timetable that personally fits you. Your body will recognize the respect you are giving it and do its very best for you.

ADVANCED-DEGREE PC

Once you have worked up to twenty flex repetitions three times a day for a week, you're ready for the next level of PC fitness.

In addition to your twenty flexes, three times a day, add in ten slow repetitions that go like this: Gradually tense the PC muscle for five seconds, hold for another five, and release for a last count of five. You should be able to feel your PC muscle slowly push in and then push out. Try doing two of these to start, three times a day, and work up to ten of them (in addition to your twenty fast flexes). It may sound simple as I've described it, but it does take a good deal of stamina so allow yourself at a minimum two to three weeks to work up to the full complement.

I cannot overemphasize the contribution these beginning and advanced PC muscle exercises make not only to sexual pleasure but also to pelvic-genital health. So please, place the work you are doing in a total, lifetime context and continue to do your flexes along with other practices of good personal self-care and hygiene on a daily basis.

LET YOUR FINGERS DO THE WALKING

Now that you are confident in your ability to identify your PC muscle and have brought it to a new level of strength and tone, you are ready to acclimate the PC muscle to flexing and relaxing in the presence of an object in your vagina.

As I mentioned earlier, many women are not able to maintain control over their PC muscle so that they can have an orgasm in the presence of a penis, dildo, or other object in the vagina. In the next series of exercises, you will insert objects into your vagina in order to build more strength and a greater sense of control. On your SSO quest it is important to know that you are physiologically in charge and in control of what is happening in your genital area during intercourse.

Now don't get me wrong. You will not be required to

be "on duty" during intercourse in the future, surveying the territory to make sure your body is functioning according to plan. The whole point of these exercises is to make the feel and activity of your toned PC and uterine muscles so comfortable and recognizable to you that when you are with your partner you will not be thinking but rather will be experiencing everything in the realm of the senses. Let's borrow a phrase from the world of dance and say we are working to train your sense memory here. Once the imprint is set you will be able to move into ecstasy without thinking about a thing. So let's get on with this intimate dance right now!

You want to start this next exercise and every exercise that follows in this chapter with the sensate focus genital caress you learned at the beginning of the chapter. Some women prefer to preface each exercise by doing a full-body caress, using oils, lotions, or baby powder, working their way slowly toward the genital area. The thing I like about this approach is that it puts each exercise in a full-body context. And that is what you want to remember at all times. This is not a sexual fix-it book nor is the aim of these chapters how to do "it" quicker, faster, better. What I am hoping to bring you is thoughtful, heartfelt information, instruction, and support to help you enrich yourself sexually one hundred percent, drawing on your own inherent sensual body beauty and intimate orgasmic power.

Relax. Lie on your back, sit up, use whatever position allows you to breathe easily, deeply, and restfully. Making sure you

*have cleaned your hands in advance and are not wearing any
perfume, rings, or bracelets that will slide up and down your
arm, insert the tip of your little finger into your vagina just one-
half of an inch (about one knuckle's worth). Sensuously
tighten your PC muscle around your fingertip and then relax it
again, just as you did the flex and release in the previous
exercises. Do twenty repetitions in this manner. See if you can
insert your fingertip up to an inch (up to the second knuckle).
Again, tighten and then release the PC muscle twenty times.
Now see if you can insert your finger all the way up to the last
knuckle. Again, flex and release for a series of twenty flexes.*

*Work your way in this three phase per finger process through
each finger on your hand. If at any time you get nervous, stop,
focus on your belly breathing, remind yourself that what you
are doing is good and natural, and see if you can start again. If
you feel pain or if these actions stimulate any fears or
uncomfortable memories you might have of an incident in your
past, stop immediately and do not start again until you have
consulted with a physician, a therapist, or both.*

BABES IN SEXUAL TOYLAND

Before I started working as a professional sexual surrogate in the early 1980s, I had never used, let alone seen,
a dildo. And neither had many of my surrogate peers, or
nonsurrogate peers for that matter. Times have changed,
however, and dildos, vibrators, and other sex toys are a
part of many women's sexual lives. I don't want to
assume, however, that they have become part of yours so

I am going to take this opportunity to tell you about them. This is not a digression though, because afterward you are going to proceed with your exercises, this time incorporating the use of a dildo into your learning plan.

When I was in high school, there was one boy in my class whose life was made a living hell because his father manufactured sex toys. I must say that while I was not one of the active participants in the teasing that continually went on, I certainly did my share of snickering. Wherever that boy is today, let me tell you now, my dear, I'm really sorry I ever laughed at you. Because what your father did, I've discovered in later years, was of immeasurable service to all of us who want to enjoy full sexual lives.

Why am I telling you this anecdote from my childhood? Well, in spite of the various sexual revolutions that have transpired since my teens, many people today still do not understand the function of items like dildos and vibrators. You can just do an informal test with people you know if you want. I guarantee you will get many giggles at the mention of the subject, along with some pretty wacky explanations of what value sex toys have in our everyday lives. Some of the misguided beliefs I've heard in my time include: (1) sex toys are for "perverts," (2) if your sex life was good you wouldn't need sex toys, and (3) using sex toys will remove the need for having sex with other people. Maybe you even believe, on some unconscious level, that one or more of these opinions are true. Let me give you some information, then, that might help you change your mind.

SHOW AND TELL

I'm going to tell you about both dildos and vibrators, even though the exercises to follow only make use of a dildo. I just think that because you may want to explore vibrators on your own, it would be good if you had some knowledge of their function and potential. Both dildos and vibrators are used to stimulate areas deep in the vagina that cannot be reached by hand. If you have never experimented with sex toys before, you will be surprised at what using them can do for you. While it is true that they can be used for individuals who are experiencing doubts, difficulties, and dilemmas about their sexuality, sex toys are a great boon to those whose sex lives are good but have the potential to become even better. Mind you, you may even hesitate to call dildos and vibrators toys because they perform so well.

A dildo is a man-made object shaped like a penis that can, but does not necessarily, vibrate. They are available in a variety of sizes. Some are made out of hard plastic but the newest models are made out of soft rubber or a gel-like substance that feels more like a real penis. They are made from molds of real penises and so have details like realistic heads and veins. The flexible kind can also be bent into different shapes. Some dildos come with the added feature of having suction cups on the base so they can be freestanding, affording women a greater variety of positions in which the dildo can be used.

For the purposes of the exercises you will be doing in this chapter I recommend you look for a dildo that:

- is shaped like a realistic penis

- is similar in size to your partner's (or the average size of the partners you have sex with)

- has a suction-cup base

- is flexible enough to be bent into a gooseneck shape to stimulate your G-spot

- vibrates at both a high and low setting (not for the purposes of this exercise, but for future use).

If you encounter difficulty finding all these attributes in one dildo, make sure that at a minimum it is realistically sized and is flexible. You might end up buying two dildos, each of which incorporates some of the attributes you are looking for. You might want to get a smaller dildo, say a four-inch one, and a larger one to work up to, particularly if you are new to using them.

A vibrator can be penis-shaped, but can come in other sizes as well; some are as tiny as a triple-A battery while others are as big as your forearm. These large vibrators are not meant to be inserted in the vagina and have instead exterior massage uses. Vibrators differ in the strength of the stimulation they provide and some contain different levels of intensity settings.

There are now many pleasant and professional stores across the country in which you can buy sex toys like dildos and vibrators. If there isn't a store near you, Appendix B contains a sample listing of mail order firms from which you can order products. I list them as a service to you, not as an endorsement. You should examine the catalogues carefully to determine if the items fit your needs and whether the prices are reasonable.

EVERYTHING OLD IS NEW AGAIN

The sensual squeezing, holding, and releasing exercise you did in the previous exercise is exactly what you are going to do in this next exercise. Only this time you are going to have a dildo in your vagina as you do the process. Start with a four-inch dildo—it can be smooth or have a pronounced head, it doesn't matter.

Now, you are not pumping iron with your PC muscle. Gentleness is the order of the day. Your aim is to accustom yourself sensually to the looseness and tightness of your PC muscle around an object inserted in your vagina. By increasing your PC muscle's sensitivity in this way, you are increasing the muscle's ability to spasm and trigger orgasm during intercourse.

Begin with a sensate focus body caress. Keep close tabs on your breathing at all times. Lubricate your dildo well. Now give yourself a genital caress with the dildo, rubbing it softly against your labia and clitoris. The first time you insert it, go only as deep as an inch. Start your PC squeezes. Squeeze, hold, release. After you have done the twenty repetitions, insert the dildo another inch and do twenty more squeezes. Insert the dildo a third inch and repeat the cycle of gentle squeezes, holds, and releases for the last time. If you start to have an orgasm, while it is not the goal of the exercise, enjoy it and keep the dildo inserted in your vagina as your PC muscle starts to spasm.

SEE G-SPOT RUN

The G-spot is not the focus of this book, yet G-spot awareness can vastly enhance your capacity for super sexual orgasm. So let's take a few moments to go over the basics here. Located on the upper wall of the vagina, about two-thirds of the way in, the G-spot feels rough to the touch. Insert a finger into your vagina and see for yourself. If you hook your finger back toward yourself and give an easy pull, you should experience a powerfully pleasurable feeling. You may find it difficult to do this maneuver, so if you don't manage to, don't worry. You will soon use a flexible dildo to achieve the effect. Before we move on with the exercise, however, let me say a few words about this much described and misdescribed facet of the female anatomy.

The G-spot is an area of extreme sensitivity for women. Stimulating it often produces an intense orgasmic response which is sometimes accompanied by an ejaculation called a "gusher." A large amount of thin, clear fluid is expelled, often running down a woman's legs in warm rivulets. The fluid is composed of a substance similar to semen but without the sperm. Contrary to old wives' tales, the fluid is definitely not urine.

Many women have had a "gusher" once and then never again for a variety of reasons:

- their partner didn't know what he did and couldn't stimulate the G-spot again

- unused to the phenomenon, the women were afraid to try the position again that stimulated the "gusher"

- unused to the phenomenon, the women consulted their physicians who told them they had lost bladder control and urinated during intercourse and advised them not to try that position again.

Let me make this unmistakably clear to you: *Having a "gusher" is an ecstatic and natural experience for every woman.*

With your new understanding of the G-spot in mind, let's now locate it using a dildo.

Start with a full sensate focus body caress. Lie on your back with your legs apart and your knees resting against your body. Take the lubricated end of the dildo gooseneck and insert it softly into your vagina. Move the dildo so that the end points toward the G-spot. Insert the dildo against the spot so that you feel a slight tug. Keep up the easy tugging motion as you tighten your vagina and the PC muscle and ever so coyly tease your G-spot by lightly pulling the dildo out of your vagina. Gradually tease your G-spot more and more by rubbing and tugging harder and harder. Stay on the edge of orgasm for as long as you can this way. Your uterine and PC muscles will gain in strength as you tease and tug. With at least an hour of weekly exercise like this you will learn how to exert a lot of pressure against the G-spot and learn to trigger a "gusher." You will also heighten the responsiveness of your PC muscle so that you can orgasm almost immediately upon penetration.

You don't have to have a "gusher" to have a super sexual orgasm, but the combination is hard to beat. So, if you're up for it, try this next G-spot exercise too.

Bend the tip of your flexible dildo and place the suction area on a flat surface. After your sensate focus warm-up, kneel or squat on top of the dildo and insert it so you are stimulating your G-spot. Increase the pressure by rubbing sensuously against the G-spot. If you are attuned, you can actually feel it swell. Now change your position so you hook the curve of the dildo into your G-spot. Thrust so that the dildo feels like a very sexy hook tugging at your G-spot. Take slow, luxurious breaths as you move toward enhanced excitement and arousal.

As you peak toward orgasm, thrust all the way down on the dildo. At this point you may experience a gushing of G-spot fluid down your legs. At the very least, you will experience a lot of lubrication, much more than you are accustomed to. With practice, this exercise can result in a fantastic guaranteed "gusher" for you.

WAITING TO EXHALE

As I'm sure you know by now, the secret to super sexual orgasm lies waiting in the cul-de-sac, the next area of focus in our sensual explorations. (It's about time!) But first, a brief review: Contrary to popular belief, the vagina does not end at the cervix and uterus but in fact continues through to the cul-de-sac (which comes from a French word meaning "bottom of the sack"). When you are not aroused, the uterus rests on top of the vagina about two-thirds of the way back, compressing the passage. When you become aroused, however, the muscles supporting the uterus can tighten, lifting the uterus up and exposing the cul-de-sac from its regular resting place behind the cervix . . . *but only if you are "SSO fit."* And now you are! So it's time to discover the cul-de-sac! Drum roll please . . .

The following exercise is designed to help you identify the cul-de-sac and the uterine muscles that, when properly controlled, will make your cul-de-sac available to you during intercourse. This exercise involves what I like to call vaginal breathing. And what you are going to do is exactly what it sounds like: inhale and exhale with your vagina. Again, may I remind you that this is a natural process derived from your body's innate functioning. As we get into the exercise, some of you may even express signs of recognition at what is going on, as you've probably felt the sensations before but just never had a name to put to them. The thing to remember is that we are not doing the exercise to experience vaginal breathing per se. The breathing is an indication that your muscles are flexing and releasing properly in order to allow your cul-de-sac to open when you want it to during intercourse.

Again, starting from a place of relaxation and ease, lie on your back with your knees bent toward and against your body as far as they will comfortably go. If you prefer to keep your knees up and your feet flat on the floor, that is fine too. When you are settled, tighten your PC muscle. Find your lower abdominal muscles—I call them uterine muscles because you can feel their placement above your uterus—and tighten them along with your PC. As you tighten, visualize yourself inhaling air into your vagina. Hold for a few seconds and then visualize yourself releasing the air in a full and complete exhale. Repeat this several times. Rest. Then repeat again. As with the PC muscle exercises, do a series of gentle repetitions the first week and then build week by week toward a regimen of twenty repetitions three times a day. You can feel, as you lie on your back and tighten your PC and uterine muscles, a squeezing in your lower abdomen. This squeezing and releasing is the secret to cul-de-sac availability.

Now, understand, this may not be an easy exercise for you to master all at once so do not become frustrated or impatient. We are dealing with subtleties here and you have to allow yourself the space, time, and, most important, opportunity to learn. If you are just not feeling that you can inhale and exhale through your vagina, try this: Do a variation on a shoulder-stand by positioning your head and elbows on the floor with your rear end angled upward. When you have gotten there, move yourself immediately out of this position and down onto your back. Do you experience a rush of air out of your vagina? This is the sensation you are going to stimulate with the tightening and releasing of the PC and uterine muscles simultaneously. Now try lying on your back again and flexing and releasing the PC and uterine muscles gently and steadily.

ALL TOGETHER NOW . . .

You are now ready to put all you've learned so far in this chapter together into one single sensuous exercise, complete with cul-de-sac penetration. This is a turning-point exercise, so prepare.

Ready yourself with an entire, languidly erotic full-body sensate focus caress. Lubricate your flexible dildo and use it to begin a genital caress. Take extra time with your genital caress and make sure to play with your PC muscle and G-spot, although not to the point of having a "gusher."

Making sure your knees and feet are in a comfortable position you identified for yourself in the previous exercise, gently insert the dildo beyond the G-spot and into the end of the vagina. To find the cervix, move the dildo until you feel it rub against the knobby surface that yields a cramping sensation. Explore the cervix to find how hard you can thrust against it or if you enjoy sensations in that area at all.

Now, as if you were having intercourse, thrust the dildo into yourself and, at the same time, flex your PC and uterine muscles simultaneously. The extra one-half to three-quarters of an inch of the cul-de-sac will open to penetration, and then close off around the dildo. Don't panic, it is not stuck there and you can always pull it out. But feel how with a light tug it still stays in position. Keep that pressure on the dildo as you keep your tugs gentle. With practice, you will be able to tighten your muscles so that you can tug harder on the dildo without pulling it out. Explore the wonder of sensations and feelings this new territory of your very own undiscovered body gives you.

Don't be surprised if your body explodes into a dramatic climax at the completion of this exercise. After all, you have penetrated the cul-de-sac. But don't feel let down if that doesn't happen. While some women will have an explosive orgasm from dildo penetration, the majority will not . . . not yet. Your body is still adjusting, and your training is not complete. Still, the sensations from this exercise are going to be incredible. So enjoy them.

A more challenging, but extremely fulfilling, variation on this exercise involves working with a dildo with a suction base. Give it a try.

After starting with a sensate focus body and genital caress, attach the suction-cup base of your lubricated dildo to a clean, smooth surface and lower yourself onto it bit by bit. Play with your PC muscle by moving up and down on the dildo as you flex, hold, and release. Lower yourself far enough now to have the dildo rub and then tug against your G-spot. You may need to curve the head of the dildo to do this. See if you can stimulate it without going all the way to a "gusher." Now stimulate the cervix with the dildo and then move on to tightening the PC and uterine muscles simultaneously as you slide the dildo all the way into the cul-de-sac. Let the cul-de-sac latch on to the dildo and move gently up and down on it,

feeling the gentle thrusting motions as the dildo tugs against the
pull of the cul-de-sac. Enjoy the pure physical delight of it all.

Please understand that from this position, it is more difficult to make the cul-de-sac available. But with practice, kindness, and patience you will get there. Don't pressure yourself to "do it right" the first time. Don't look to have an orgasm. And certainly don't look to have a super sexual orgasm. Just explore your reactions and value whatever experiences come your way. Take as long as you like and repeat both of these cul-de-sac exercises a few times each week before moving on to the next chapter.

3

Motion

ou may not know where you've heard the expression, but I'm sure you've heard it somewhere: "It's not the meat, it's the motion." Now these words may make you blush; you may find them a little crude or naughty or nasty. But somewhere inside of you, I know these words also ring totally true. Motion is exactly what we are going to be talking about in this chapter, the enticingly pleasurable dance of sexual connection that is so crucial for making a super sexual orgasm connection.

Rhythm, timing, pacing, position: You didn't realize there were that many details and fine points to the experience of lovemaking, did you? That's okay. You're not the only one. The majority of people do not understand the primary importance each of these elements plays in the enjoyment of an intimate encounter, let alone an SSO encounter. But they are *all* important.

It's a fact: Even the most gorgeous people do not make for gorgeous lovemaking if those people are out of sync or in the wrong place at the wrong time. And you can have all the moves and grooves down to a *T*, but if the approach is off-speed, your bang will turn into a bust. But we're not going to let that happen. You *are* going to reach your goal of super sexual orgasm. You just need to first learn a little bit about the motions that will get you there.

WALK DON'T RUN

Most people think good sex is fast and riotously turbulent: slam bam, thank you ma'am. That's the way it's portrayed in the media, right? Well, it is true that good sex can sometimes be fast. And I certainly would give my eye-tooth to have been a part of some of the passionately breakneck rendezvous I've watched on the silver screen. However, in the real world, the most luxurious, excruciatingly delightful, nerve-tingling, explosively fulfilling, shimmering cascades-of-lights-flashing-behind-the-eyes sex grows out of an approach that is *slow*, *focused*, and *caressing*. The greatest orgasmic payoffs come from moving your body symbiotically with your partner's body—gently, undulatingly, and sinuously. And if these adverbs don't seem to apply to you or the one you love, don't despair. We're going to change all that with the simple exercises you are about to learn.

In the course of this phase of your journey toward super sexual orgasm, you are going to find out how much subtle yet powerful control you can bring to the process of your own excitement and orgasm by working with the elements of rhythm, timing, and pacing. You are going to learn every facet of what makes you aroused, how to escalate your pleasure increment by increment, adjust it in keeping with your partner's arousal if you want to, and then finally, when you are ready, find release through orgasm. You are going to practice working with your motion and energy so that your union will be as satisfying as possible. And you are going to learn about how to best position your body during lovemaking in order to engage every muscle and sinew into your hypnotic sexual dance.

You are about to enter the advanced circle of lovemaking knowledge that will ensure that each one of your liaisons will be fantastic, always different, and continuously surprising. You will be able to magnificently satisfy yourself and your partner every time and every moment you make love. To borrow a little lingo from the world of television, once you have moved into this advanced circle of lovemaking knowledge, there will be no more repeats for you, only original sexual programming.

Let's start developing your show right now.

PLACES EVERYONE

In real estate, they say the three most important things are location, location, location. To achieve a cul-de-sac

SSO, the three most important things are position, position, position. If this sends you into a tailspin of concern that you aren't up to swinging from the chandeliers or doing the wild thing on the top of a pool table, *stop worrying now*. It's all much more simple than you imagined. And when you experience the results, well, you might just be jazzed enough to hop on the nearest chandelier. (You go, girl!)

Here's a news flash: When it comes to super sexual orgasm, all intercourse positions are not the same. Certain positions are far more likely to provide the stimulation you need to have an SSO. You have your preferences of course, and I don't want to dissuade you from continuing to enjoy them. Just know that it will be much more difficult to have the cul-de-sac open in all but the positions I am about to describe.

But first, another news flash: The missionary style of intercourse is the position *least* likely to bring a woman to climax (which would account for why so many woman describe their sexual lives as only moderately pleasurable). The problem with the missionary position, more than anything, is a motion problem. In this classic sexual position, where the woman lies with her legs straight out and her partner lies on top of her, it is difficult, if not impossible, for a woman to move her pelvis. The only way she can thrust is to tense her leg muscles, and this tension prevents her from relaxing into arousal. Limited motion means limited feeling, and that means limited pleasure.

You are already working very hard to complete many

new exercises and learn new techniques. You want this hard work to pay off, and that payoff might not happen if your intercourse position is working *against* your SSO.

KICK UP YOUR HEELS

Your mission, should you decide to accept it, is to transcend the missionary position and head for more fertile ground. Bear with me for a moment and put aside everything you've ever heard of or experienced about the physical positions of lovemaking. I am going to tell you now about a lovemaking position very few people practice, not because it is difficult or bizarre, but because it's so simple—people just tend to overlook it. Yet this position is your ticket to transcendence, providing you and your lover the best possible alignment of your bodies to consistently achieve SSO.

The intercourse position I recommend starts with you lying on your back with your knees bent and your legs up in the air. Your partner will kneel between your legs using his knees to support his weight (this is very important, as it keeps you more free to move). You can rest your legs on your partner's shoulders or you can have your calves rest against your thighs. In this configuration, penetration will stimulate your PC muscle, G-spot, cervix, and cul-de-sac. The kneeling position also allows for the deepest penetration by the man. In this position, he can always also withdraw his penis and use it to stimulate your clitoris and urethra.

This position takes a little getting used to, but once

you are comfortable with it, you will be amazed at how powerful, confident, sensitized, and sexy you will feel. You may want to introduce this new position to your partner the next time you are making love. This will give you both ample opportunity to get comfortable with the position before setting your sights on your first super sexual orgasm.

THE MISSIONARY RIDES AGAIN!

Now at first, some of you just may not be able to give up the missionary position in favor of the alternative I just described. If you are a devotee of the missionary life, here is a subtle adjustment you can make to that traditional position that will significantly increase your chances of having a gratifying orgasm.

Once your partner has inserted his erect penis into you as he normally would in intercourse in the missionary position, your partner will move his entire body up on top of you about two inches. He will be, as they say, "riding high." Your partner's pubic bone will rest above yours so that the base of his penis presses against your clitoris. This provides a sensuously continuous stimulation of the clitoris during intercourse.

The type of thrusting done in this "riding high" position is actually very slight, more like gentle, surging, circular motions. Your pelvises will move, but the rest of your bodies will not. And since your bodies' range of motion is restricted, you will tire less quickly and can continue your lovemaking well into the day or night.

AROUSAL BY NUMBERS

In order to achieve SSO, you need to marshal all your sexual energies. And in order to do this, you have to be intimately familiar with your personal process of arousal. We will explore the concepts of peaking and platcauing—first going solo, with only you doing the exercises, and then with your partner—as a means of deciphering the exciting mysteries of your personal sexual arousal script.

Now, I caution you, this is the part of the learning process that may seem especially mechanical at first because you are having to actively think about what you are feeling instead of just feeling it. And there is also an "arousal scale" that you will need to keep in mind (more on that in a moment). Just trust me that once you understand the workings of your arousal, all the mechanics will dissolve and you will be left with a healthy knowledge of what makes you feel good and the ability to bring yourself that pleasure every time you make love.

Think of your levels of sexual arousal on a scale from 1 to 10. On this scale, level 1 is no arousal and level 10 is orgasm. A twinging feeling in the genital area will be 2 or 3 while 4 is a steady low level of arousal. When you are at 5 or 6 you are in the medium range and by 7 and 8 your heart will pound and you might be slightly short of breath. At 9 you are just on the precipice before orgasm, and at 10 you have reached your climax.

Please understand this is not a *performance* scale but rather a *magnitude* scale that will give you a means of tracking the intensity of your arousal. Your 1 and your 10 will be different from everyone else's. So just give up thinking in terms of comparisons and concentrate on yourself.

CLIMB EVERY MOUNTAIN

You are now going to explore what arousal means to you through the process known as peaking. You will caress your own genitals and learn to modulate your arousal so that it goes up and down in a series of peaks that are under your control. In this first exercise, and all the exercises to follow, you are going to want to make sure you have at least one hour of quiet time, in an interruption-free environment.

Begin a slow sensate focus genital caress, paying close attention to the point of contact. Make sure to breathe and to relax all your muscles. Keep asking yourself what arousal level you feel you are at as the caressing continues. Do not try to reach a particular level of arousal. Just note what you are feeling and make your best guess where that would be on the arousal scale of 1 to 10.

Go slowly. Be gentle with yourself. Keep your fingers, wrists, and arms supple. If your attention drifts, consistently bring it back to the sensations you are feeling at the point of contact. If at the end of this exercise you want to have an orgasm, go ahead.

In this next exercise, you will actually peak.

Start your slow sensate focus genital caress. Caress your genitals past the twinging stage (level 3). Then stop the stimulation and allow yourself to drop back to arousal level 1. Start caressing

yourself again, and this time go up to level 5. Stop the stimula-
tion again and allow your arousal to drop a couple of levels.
Repeat this cycle, each time taking your peak to a new level, all
the way up to level 9. Try to make each cycle of peaking and
dropping last for five minutes. You can conclude the exercise
with an orgasm if you like but it is not mandatory.

Repeat this peaking exercise once or twice a week until
you feel you have a good measure of control over your
arousal. I want you to be loving to yourself during these
exercises. This is very intimate, personal work you are
doing. Be patient with yourself and resist the temptation
to just caress yourself straight to orgasm. You may find
that with practice, your orgasms are becoming stronger.
The whole process, you see, engages, charges, and
focuses your sexual energies, which are essential to SSO.

FROM THE MOUNTAINS TO THE VALLEYS

Now that you have mastered the art of peaking you are
ready for plateauing. Plateauing is just like peaking
except that you hover at each level of arousal for a while,
creating a plateau. Remember to take your time. Do
each exercise for three weeks if that's what it takes for
you to get comfortable with the process. And enjoy yourself. Let yourself be in the right frame of mind to get the
art of plateauing under your belt.

Start this exercise, as you have started all the exercises in this
chapter, with a sensuous genital self-caress. Relax your muscles

and take long, luxurious breaths. Comfortably allow your arousal to go to level 4 and try to stay at this level for thirty seconds. Bring yourself to just above 4. Slowly take two deep belly breaths. This will allow your arousal level to go down. Let it go to 3 and then start to accelerate your breathing till you pant so as to increase your arousal level back up toward 4. Hover between 3 and 4 for thirty seconds or more just by speeding up your breathing.

Repeat this exercise several times, each time choosing an increasingly higher plateau level to reach and then drop from. If you find the higher levels are difficult for you, focus your attention on the highest level you can comfortably plateau at for at least a week. Then try a higher level. You will find that with increasing body awareness, focusing, breath work, and muscle strength, plateauing at the higher levels will become natural and comfortable for you.

ROCK ON

In this exercise you will adjust your arousal level through pelvic movements. The basic principle is that greater movement will heighten arousal while decreased movement will tone levels back down. Having a flexible pelvis is advantageous well beyond the purposes of this exercise, though. Such flexibility is good for your back, as it takes the stress out of pelvic muscles, hips, thighs, and buttocks. You will be able to comfortably do more sexual positions, and, as you will find out here, greater flexibility will enable you to become more aroused. *Too much tension in the pelvic area compromises sensations of sexual pleasure.*

Before you proceed through this exercise, however, you need to learn the basics of pelvic motion: thrusts and rolls.

Pelvic thrusts can be done standing up or lying down. If you choose to stand, plant your feet shoulder-width apart. Gently but firmly rock your pelvis from back to front without moving any other parts of your body. Don't wiggle your butt or shimmy your hips. Just tilt your pelvis twenty times.

If you do the thrusts lying down, put your knees up and rock your buttocks slowly up and down so they are the only part of you that moves off the floor. Keep your other muscles relaxed and keep your pace even and slow.

Pelvic rolls can also be done lying down. The roll is a continuous, sensuous motion of the hips. It may help you to imagine that you are using a hula hoop. If you want to actually get a hoop to practice with, that's fine. Do a series of rolls at different speeds and especially spend time doing long, liquid rolls.

Once you have gotten the feel of the thrusts and rolls, combine the motions for at least ten minutes a day. Put on some music, close your eyes, and let every molecule in your body get into the groove.

Now let's get to the arousal modulation exercise through pelvic motion.

Caress yourself to level 3 or 4. At this point, start in with the pelvic rolls and thrusting, alternating gently between the two movements. Even though you are by yourself, make each of your movements as sensual and alluring as possible. Allow your arousal to increase to level 6 and then slow or stop the pelvic action till your arousal drops below 6. Start the rolls and thrusts again till you push up above level 6. Plateau there for at least thirty seconds. Repeat this exercise every day till you feel comfortable regulating your arousal levels in this manner.

BAIT AND SWITCH

During sexual activity it is possible to focus on many things that are going on. In the previous exercise, for instance, I had you focus on the pelvic area and the sensations of arousal the thrusts and rolls evoked. Now in this next exercise, you are going to touch one area while focusing on another, the aim being to use this change in focus to maintain an arousal plateau.

Sensuously caress your genitals until you reach level 6. Slowly continue to caress yourself until you feel you have edged just past this point. While you continue to stroke a particular genital area, switch your mental focus to a different genital area that you are not currently touching. For instance, if you are rubbing your clitoris, continue to touch it, but focus on the sensations you are experiencing in your inner vaginal lips. Your arousal level will decrease. When it reaches 5, switch your focus back to the area you are caressing and bring your arousal back up to level 6. See if you can plateau here for thirty seconds

*by switching your focus as you previously did from the place
where you were touching yourself to another part of your genital
area.*

*Once you are comfortable with this technique, you will be
able to use it to plateau at any level you choose.*

THE MAIN SQUEEZE

The final plateauing method you are going to learn
involves the PC muscle. Since you have been working
out daily it should be in excellent shape.

*Begin with your sensuous genital caress. Caress yourself slowly
until you reach a point just beyond level 7. Take your time
getting there. Enjoy your experiences, breathe, and relax. When
you arrive, squeeze your PC muscle a couple of times. Do you
notice your arousal level drops each time you squeeze? Keep
squeezing till you drop below 6 and then plateau there for
thirty seconds. Start caressing your way back up to 7. Repeat
the squeezing process to bring yourself down to 6, plateau
there, and then bring your arousal up to 7 again.*

Imagine that . . . now you know *four* different methods
for plateauing. Try combining them, using different con-
figurations to modulate your plateauing. With practice
you will be able to use all of them to stay at high levels of
arousal for several minutes. Again, remember to allow
yourself enough time to understand in a deep, body
sense how all these methods work. You don't want to
gloss over these techniques—they will provide an essen-

tial foundation for the SSO experience coming up in the next chapter.

TWO FOR THE AROUSAL ROAD

You are now ready to move on to arousal control exercises that you and your partner can do together. But before we begin, we need to take a moment to introduce your partner to the sensate focus caress.

To ensure you are clearly communicating the important elements to your partner, let me summarize by saying that sensate focus is:

- Slow: Whatever speed you think is slow, cut it in half and you will much better approximate the true level of slowness appropriate to sensate focus touching.

- Pressure-free: There is no demand here to perform or achieve a result for you or your partner. There is no aim other than the caress itself and the person caressing is only required to pleasure him- or herself.

- Focused: Pay attention to the temperature, texture, contrast, and shape of what you touch. If you become distracted, bring your mind back to focusing on the point of touch and sensations associated with this.

- Present: Touching takes place in the here and now. Past and future are not relevant. Be fully in every moment of touch.

- Sensuous: Experience the pure, uninhibited pleasure of skin stroking against skin.

Whenever you do a sensate focus caress with a partner, one of you will be taking an *active* role and one of you will be taking a *passive* role. The active partner is the one doing the caressing; the passive partner is the recipient of the caress, whose only "job" is to relax and enjoy the experience. You will switch roles for some of these exercises, so don't be concerned about who goes first. Again, please understand there is no issue of performance or skill involved in the exercises. The only purpose is pleasure, and whether you are the active partner or the passive one, you are focusing on your own good feelings (of course, never in a way that makes your partner uncomfortable).

In this next exercise, your partner is going to learn about sensate focus from your loving example, and then get a chance to practice what he has learned. Before you begin, be certain that both of you have at least forty-five minutes of time to set aside for each other.

To begin this exercise your partner will lie comfortably on his back with his legs spread slightly apart. His arms can be at his sides or under his head.

Lie at your partner's side, making as much body contact as possible. Slowly begin to give your lover a full-body caress, starting with the face, neck, shoulders, and arms. Move down to the chest, stomach, and genitals, and then farther down to the thighs, calves, feet, and toes. Make this a fluid progression from head to toe, avoiding choppy transitions that may startle him.

After fifteen minutes of full-body caressing, it is time to give your lover the experience of a genital caress. Using lots of baby oil or other sensuous lubricant, shift the focus of your caress now exclusively to your partner's genitals. Slowly caress the penis and scrotum. Move your fingers around the shaft and head of the penis. Run your fingers around each testicle. But don't focus on turning your partner on. Feel good yourself. Look at his genitals closely and see what they do—how they change texture, shape, and color when they are relaxed and when they are aroused. Take this opportunity to learn every centimeter of your partner's gorgeous gifts.

Now it is time to switch roles. Your partner will begin by giving you a slow, sensuous full-body caress, mimicking the techniques he just learned from you. Allow him to explore with his hands from top to bottom, always keeping a point of contact with your body, and keeping focused on that point of contact.

After fifteen minutes of this full-body caress, your partner is ready to begin a genital caress. As your partner explores your genitals, encourage him to feel the warmth and texture of your outer vaginal lips, inner lips, perineum, clitoris, and vaginal walls. Luxuriate in the sensations of his caress.

At the conclusion of this exercise, give your partner feedback on the experience. If his movements were too quick, rough, or anxious, let him know now. Then set aside a time to go through this exercise again. You both need to feel very good about what you are experiencing together before you move on to more complex exercises.

And please note: If disquieting emotional material comes up for you (or for your partner) during these exercises or you feel in any way physically compromised, whether you understand why or not, immediately cease the activity. Explain to your partner that this area is problematic for you. A partner who is really there for you will not be offended or take it personally, but rather will be totally respectful of your experience and support your choice to explore what you are feeling with a doctor or therapist.

PARTNERS IN PLEASURE

Now that your partner has learned about sensate focus, you are truly ready for the next level of arousal exercises. Let's begin with an awareness exercise to get you used to interacting with your partner and communicating your levels of arousal. You will need to set a time in advance for this exercise—a time when you will both be committed to spending a full hour together, free of distractions and interruptions.

Lie on your back comfortably with your arms and legs slightly spread. Have your partner lie down beside you and begin a sensuous body caress, gradually moving down to your genitals. Your partner should then start a slow genital caress, perhaps intermixing it with sensuous oral sex. His tongue should gently but urgently stroke your vulva and clitoris. Every few minutes or so your partner should ask you your arousal level. Let him know what your level is each time he asks, yet try to keep your focus on your mounting pleasure as he continues the caressing and oral sex.

It does not matter how high your arousal goes or whether it fluctuates. The important thing for you is to recognize what levels you are at when you are being stimulated by another person, and to be able to communicate this information clearly to that person. Don't be shy about saying what you are feeling, whether it's the tiniest twinge or the most compelling cataclysm. And remember, if you are brought to orgasm, enjoy it. But keep in mind that it is a benefit, not a goal.

When you have completed the exercise, you may want to switch roles and give your partner a chance to practice his communication skills as the passive partner.

HIGH AND MIGHTY

In this next partner exercise, you are going to explore peaking, with your partner playing the active role.

Again, you will lie on your back with your arms and legs spread slightly. Have your partner start a front caress and gradually move to your genitals. He will caress these ever so slowly, and then gently spread your legs so he can see your inner vaginal lips. Your lover will then lick from the bottom of your vaginal opening up the center of your vaginal lips with the tip of the tongue, gliding over your clitoris on the way upward to the top.

Use all of your attention and focus to sense the path his tongue takes. Your partner should do this licking several times, each more slowly than the last. In addition, your lover can also insert the tip of a finger into your vagina and delicately stroke the muscles around your vaginal opening. This may make the PC muscle spasm as it tightens around his finger.

When you reach level 3, tell your partner you are at 3 and ask him to stop caressing till your arousal drops a few levels. Really notice what happens throughout your body as your arousal drops. Then ask your partner to commence caressing again.

Repeat this arousal process so that you peak at levels 5 through 9, backing off two levels each time before continuing. Remember to focus on the point of contact. Breathe and relax your muscles. You may climax during this exercise. If you do, try to stay as passive as possible. Some amount of involuntary muscle tension will occur. However, the more passive you remain, the more familiar you will become with how your body feels during high arousal levels and orgasm.

If you do not go very high up the first few times you do this peaking exercise, don't worry, this will change with practice. You have done what you needed to do just by recognizing the arousal levels you have reached and communicating this to your partner. And remember, the sensations associated with the downcurve of a sexual peak are as important to familiarize yourself with as the feelings you have on the upswing. Also, please feel comfortable repeating this exercise as many times as you and your partner like. Switch roles if you wish. And don't forget to keep up with your *solo* peaking and plateauing exercises on a weekly basis.

LEVEL BEST

In this next exercise, plateauing with a partner, you are going to use all those techniques you used in the solo plateauing process, so you might want to review them now. Recall that plateauing involved the PC muscle, breathing, pelvic thrusts and rolls, and focus switching. Once again, your partner will be taking the active role.

Start as before by lying on your back with your arms and legs slightly spread. Your partner will do a slow front caress before moving to your genitals. Have your partner get your arousal level up to 5 by oral sex. Your lover can maintain the stimulation throughout this exercise by use of hands, fingers, lips, and tongue.

Plateau at level 5 by regulating your breathing, push a little past 5, and then drop back below 5. Take yourself above 5 again by panting, move on to level 6, and plateau there by using your PC muscle. Squeeze your PC to drop yourself below 6 and then take yourself higher. Maintain the higher plateau through pelvic thrusts and rolls.

Start mixing it all up to see, for instance, if PC muscle relaxation in concert with thrusts gives you more or less plateau control. In other words, start experimenting with the array of techniques before you. If you are up to it, see if you can use all of the plateauing methods at the same time.

PLUNGING AHEAD

If you can successfully plateau at levels 7 and 8, you are ready for this next exercise, which involves penetration partner peaking—try saying that three times fast! Before you begin, make sure to have a vaginal lubricant handy. And note too that though your partner has the active role in this exercise, you may have to provide him with some manual and/or oral stimulation during the exercise so that he can be aroused enough to kneel over you and penetrate you at the appropriate time.

Have your partner begin a front caress with you, and slowly, slowly move down to caressing your genitals. Let him manually and orally stimulate you till you peak to level 5.

Now bend your legs and raise them in the air. You can leave them suspended or rest your calves against your thighs. Have your partner kneel between your legs with his genitals up against yours—this is the optimal position for having an SSO, remember? Your partner will gently rub his penis up against your vaginal lips in the same upward motion he used with his tongue during the peaking exercise. You will feel your clitoris twinge as he slowly glides over it with his penis.

Remember, both of you: focus, breathe, and relax.

At this point, your partner will apply lubricant to your vagina and to his penis. He will then insert just the head of the penis into your vagina. Peak to 6 while the head of your lover's penis stimulates your PC muscle.

Your partner will then insert his penis all the way into your vagina as slowly as possible. Both of you, stay focused and relaxed and open to the gentle, circling, and in and out motion of the penis in the vagina. The goal is concentration, not excitement, though you may feel that the latter is the way to go.

Your partner will continue to caress the inside of your vagina with his penis as sensuously as possible. You may want to think of his penis as a giant tongue that is licking the inside of your vagina. If your partner's penis has a curve to it, see if you can sense it brushing against your G-spot and making it swell. You may feel breathless, but make sure to breathe.

You will find that you can peak at levels up to 9 with this type of stimulation. If you want to peak all the way to orgasm, go ahead. You may even have multiple orgasms. But be sure you are not rushing toward this release. The goal of this exercise is a steady, slow build of peaks.

RISE AND SHINE

In this final exercise your partner will again be the active one while you concentrate on achieving an increasing series of plateaus. As before, make sure you have lubricant handy and prepare to stimulate your lover before you lie down for your sensuous caress.

Have your partner excite you through manual and oral stimulation to a peak at level 5. Then, as in the previous exercise, put your legs up in the air and bend your knees. Your partner will kneel between your legs and put lubricant on his penis and on your vagina. Slowly, he will start to caress the outside of your genitals before moving on to insert the head and then the shaft of his penis inside of you.

As your partner moves in gentle, swirling strokes, see if you *can plateau at levels 6 through 9 using the plateauing techniques you are familiar with: PC squeezing, breathing, pelvic movements, and switching focus. Combine the methods once you have tried them out individually at least three times. Try to plateau at level 9 for as long as you can and then let yourself fall over the edge into orgasm.*

Take your time with each plateau and make sure when you are there to inform your partner about where you are and what you are feeling. The more you communicate your sensations, the better the sex with your lover will be.

If the ecstasy of these exercises was pretty terrific, wait till you get to the next chapter. You'll be drawing on everything you've learned so far so that you can escalate your pleasure into your first super sexual orgasm. Explosive sex here you come!

4

Control

You've arrived. It's time to integrate all you have learned to produce the ultimate erotic pay-off for a woman: super sexual orgasm!

In this chapter we will bring it all together—the exercises, the techniques, the positions, the motion, the mental attitude, the works—and experience all of the magic of super sexual orgasm for the first time during lovemaking. That was some long sentence! And you might be thinking, hold on—that's a lot of stuff to be on top of at a time when you most want to be giving over everything to your senses.

I'm not going to kid you. There is some effort required at first. It will probably take a small amount of practice to coordinate various muscles and movements, and some awkwardness is to be expected. But it's a lot simpler than you might imagine. And any woman who has completed the exercises in this book thus far has *everything* she needs to experience *total control*, and to experience the ultimate pleasure of super sexual orgasm.

Total control yields total pleasure. But it is pleasure to be shared. Having control does not mean that your partner will become an incidental element in the process, a barely useful appendage just along for the ride. To the contrary, with total control, intimacy is heightened because the woman is not dependent on the man for accessing her sexual pleasure. She is offering everything she has in her sensual being to pleasure them both. When two individuals who fully embody the peak capacity of their sexuality meet, it's the stuff of fireworks and dreams. And when you give yourself over to your own super sexual orgasm, all this will be your reality.

READY ... SET ...

Before we get to the exercises where you actually experience penetration into the cul-de-sac for a super sexual orgasm, we need to do a series of partner-accompanied warm-ups with your old friends, peaking and plateauing. The difference this time is that, unlike the previous peaking and plateauing partner exercises you learned in

Chapter 3, *you* will be the active partner. This time the control is in your hands—and body—completely. See how much you enjoy this kind of experience!

You need to give yourselves at least one hour for each of these exercises. And, as before, you need to choose a comfortable environment where you will not be interrupted.

Your partner should understand that throughout these exercises he is to remain passive and relaxed at all times, communicating only if something happens that is uncomfortable or painful.

Pleasure your lover with a front caress, followed by a sensuous genital caress. Continue with an oral caress if this feels good to both of you. Do all of this slowly and sensuously, remembering that every moment of this experience is to be savored by both of you.

When your lover gets an erection, gently kneel on top of him and start to caress your genitals with his penis in the same way he caressed you in the exercises in the previous chapter. Peak through low and medium arousal levels as you stroke your vaginal lips and clitoris with his penis. Explore all kinds of touches. Move your body intuitively. Pleasure yourself in any way you feel you want to, as long as it is not painful to your lover.

When you feel ready, insert the head of your partner's penis into your vagina and squeeze and release your PC muscle luxuriously and orgiastically. See if you can peak to level 7 a few times by doing this.

Are you relaxed? Breathing deeply? Focused on the sensations of the moment? Good, then you are ready to lower yourself all the way so that your partner's penis is fully inside of you.

Remember the way you explored every inch of your vagina with a dildo? Do the same thing with your mate's penis now, fluidly moving up and gently down along your lover's shaft. Tune in to the needs of your body. If you feel like doing something, don't hold back. Put it into action. See if you can peak this way several times to level 8.

Use long, sinuous thrusts. Allow your lover's penis to go all the way in and all the way out. If you have strong leg muscles, you can actually squat as you do this. (If you want to build up this strength, you can always practice with a dildo as well.) I have also found that the more athletic the person, the more easily she can accomplish such squatting maneuvers—skiers seem especially adept. Resting some of your weight on the palms of your hands will also enable you to use your arm strength to move yourself up and down on your partner's penis.

Peak at level 9 a few times and then let yourself fall over the edge into orgasm. At the moment before you come, open your eyes, take a deep breath, and stop thrusting. Passively experience your orgasm. That is to say, just allow it to happen. Feel your PC muscle spasm around your lover's shaft. Your orgasm will be a series of shivers or spasms which may include not only your PC muscle but also your arms, legs, and facial muscles. This is not a super sexual orgasm, though it should still feel pretty intense.

I like to suggest to women that they do this exercise while focusing each time on a specific orgasm trigger. For example, you might do one whole set of increasing peaks while you zero in on stimulating your G-spot. Then you might change focus to the PC muscle, and after that, the cul-de-sac. The point here is giving you, the woman, the option of how you want to be stimulated and when. It is a revelation like no other to discover that you do indeed have this power.

You can put an exciting spin on the exercise you just completed by changing the way you thrust on your partner's penis when all of it is inside you. First, kneel over your partner and lie against his chest. Support yourself on your elbows and keep your buttocks as high in the air as possible while still keeping his penis inside of you. This will put his penis in contact with your G-spot. Now thrust sensuously back and forth. You will be able to feel your partner's penis rubbing against the spot. You may even have a "gusher."

Let's now put that pelvic rock and roll talent of yours to work. The key here is to think of yourself as moving up along your partner's penis rather than down on it. Sway your hips in a circular, undulating motion and slowly thrust your lover's penis all the way in and almost all the way out. Focus on every inch of sensation you derive from this exquisite contact. Envision this as yet another kind of oral sex, with your vagina as a mouth licking and holding your partner's hard penis.

MESA GRANDE

Once you have learned to control your peaks with your partner's penis inside of you, this ability to understand

and control your body can be used to plateau at high arousal levels with your lover for long periods of time.

As before, start with a languorous front, genital, and oral caress of your lover, who is again to remain passive and relaxed throughout. You can use either the kneeling, squatting, or lying flat techniques you just employed in the peaking exercise.

Remember the elements of successful plateauing? They are, of course, controlling your PC muscle, adjusting your breathing, changing you hip motions, and switching your focus. Work slowly and deliberately through your plateaus. Don't gloss over the lower levels. In fact, make sure you plateau at levels 4 and 5 at least twice to ensure your body is warmed up and that you are comfortable with all the plateauing techniques.

Practice plateauing at each orgasm trigger site—PC muscle, G-spot, cervix, and cul-de-sac by using your PC muscle, using your breathing, alternating your hip movements, and switching your focus. Then combine all the techniques so that you can use any variation of them at any site at any given time. As you get up to the higher levels, try to maintain your arousal levels for increasing amounts of time.

Your partner's arousal levels will climb even as he remains passive and relaxed. It will help for him to remember to breathe deeply and slowly. As you get more and more proficient with your plateauing, your partner will be able to start to move and you will not be distracted by such activity. It will strengthen the connection between you and your partner and enhance the sensuality and enjoyability of this experience if you look deeply into each other's eyes as you do this exercise.

Some of my clients have told me that they've felt an energy circling between them and their partner—going from the genitals up, through, and across their gaze and back down to the genitals again.

Now the best way to have an orgasm after your series of high-level plateaus is to reach a level 9 plateau using heavy breathing, intense pelvic thrusting, and PC muscle contractions. Then, when you are ready for an orgasm, stop everything. That's right—bring all your activity to a halt. You will tumble over into a fabulous series of involuntary orgasmic spasms.

STROKE OF LUCK

Let's try one last exercise to confirm the sense of control you have over your lovemaking before you go for your first cul-de-sac super sexual orgasm. Many women think that the longer they have intercourse, the more likely they are to have an orgasm, and many men think this is true of women too. But nothing could be further from the truth. For one thing, if you are not aroused, you won't have an orgasm regardless of how long intercourse lasts. However, if you are *very* aroused, you can have an orgasm with *a couple of strokes* of penetration from your partner. The secret to this is the control the woman exerts, not the penetration itself.

Have your partner lie on his back. Begin a front caress, continue to a genital caress, and then add oral stimulation if this pleases you both. As your partner becomes erect, generously but slowly stimulate yourself by rubbing your clitoris and vaginal lips against his penis. Don't insert it though. You may need to spend fifteen minutes or so pleasuring yourself in this manner. After your arousal is well under way, peak up to levels 7 and 8. In between your peaks, use manual or oral stimulation to help your partner maintain his high arousal levels.

Keep your leg muscles and PC muscles as relaxed as possible. Stay also in the here and now, experiencing the feelings of the moment, not anticipating what will happen down the line. Your eyes should be closed and your breathing should reach a panting level. Peak to level 9 this way. Now, as you are on the brink of orgasm, open your eyes, take a deep breath, and thrust yourself all the way down on your partner's shaft. You will likely reach orgasm within the next couple of strokes.

I cannot tell you what an exhilarating, breathtaking exercise this is. You will feel so energized and satisfied after you have done it—and secure in the knowledge that you are fully at home in your own body. Practice this technique until you can have an orgasm on the *first* stroke. In this regard, you will find that the more times you can get yourself to peak at level 9 before going into orgasm, the greater the likelihood that you will have that orgasm immediately.

You can also enhance your ability to climax on the first stroke through the use of the PC muscle. When you are at the point of opening your eyes, taking a deep breath, and thrusting yourself down, pull your PC muscle shut around your partner's shaft as well. This will often immediately trigger a powerful orgasm, especially if your PC muscle is already on the edge of a spasm.

GOING ALL THE WAY

Are you ready for the sensory experience of a lifetime? Are you ready for lights, camera, and action? Are you ready to take control? I'll bet you are. Well, here's your chance: the super sexual orgasm exercise you've been patiently waiting for. It's the big payoff. The one you have so fully earned. So go for it! Any more words will get in the way.

You want to get yourself and your partner into the mood again by doing some body caressing, genital caressing, and oral stimulation. Once you have both reached a moderate level of arousal in this fashion, take the intercourse position you've become so comfortable with: You are lying on your back with your knees bent and your legs up in the air and your partner is kneeling between your legs using his knees to support his weight. Again, you can rest your legs on your partner's shoulders or you can have your calves rest against your thighs.

Once engaged in intercourse, you are now going to slowly move through a series of increasingly higher peaks, starting at level 6. Make sure to peak at least twice at every level, always dropping back after you have achieved one peak before going on to the next. If you peak more than twice at each level, you will definitely enhance your prospects of having an SSO climax to remember.

When you have peaked at level 9 for a second time, signal your partner to thrust into you as hard as he can. As he does so, pull in your lower abdominal muscles, tighten your PC muscle, and in so doing allow your cul-de-sac to open up. Your partner's penis will slide deeper and you will grip his shaft there. Brace yourself. The sensations both of you will have will be incredible. And yours will be especially incredible because you are having your first super sexual orgasm.

If you change your breathing to panting, you can even go into a series of multiple SSOs! Your partner will feel like his orgasm is being pulled out of him. And you will feel like you are on top of the world.

Fabulous! Absolutely fabulous! A power you have never felt before. A pleasure you have never felt before. A level of ecstasy you could have never known. That's a super sexual orgasm.

You'll probably want to rest for a while now and bask in the glow of your stunning success. You should. You have truly earned it, and now it is yours forever. So savor it. Revel in it. Share a champagne toast with your partner: To SSO . . . the ultimate pleasure!

However . . . if you are one of those women who is ready to burn the midnight oil, there is one last exercise I want to share with you here to give you an SSO option. Try it now. Try it another time. But do try it.

Essentially, the intercourse position in this final exercise is the inverse of what you were using in the previous exercise. In other words, this is a cul-de-sac penetration exercise with you, the woman, *on top*.

As before, begin with a sensate focus body caress, moving on to a genital caress perhaps with some oral sex included as well. Now start to tease your vagina and clitoris with your partner's penis. After you have luxuriated in this wonderful sex play for as long as you desire, insert your lover's erect penis inside of you and start peaking slowly and suggestively through to levels 6, 7, and 8. Recall the way you used the dildo in past exercises to pleasure yourself at all excitement points when you were on top and do the same here with your partner's penis.

Plateau at level 8. After plateauing, continue to excite yourself with your partner's penis inside of you, to level 9. Be adventurous and daring with the motion of your thrusts. But make sure all the while to keep your movements as slow and sinuous as possible. Now, here's the kicker: As you plateau at level 9, lean back as far as you comfortably can, supporting yourself with your hands for balance (recall the exquisite sexual maneuver Sharon Stone performed in the movie Basic Instinct), and tighten your lower abdominal muscles while keeping your PC muscle relaxed. In this position, the cul-de-sac will now open, enabling you to push down that little bit extra on your partner's penis and grasp it there. You will cascade over into a voluptuous super sexual orgasm that you can repeat as many times as you wish. Wow!

If you had tried to experiment with this position before (after you saw the movie, perhaps), it would not have worked the same magic. Pleasurable, yes. But no SSO. Why? Because you didn't have the strength, you didn't have the motion, and you didn't have the control. But now you do. Now you have it all. You have strength, motion, position, control, and experience bringing them all together. And that adds up to the super sexual orgasm.

PLEASURE NOW, PLEASURE FOREVER

That's it. You have all the basic information and experience you need to create the ultimately intense sexual encounter with your lover. Congratulations.

Having worked hard, and followed all my instructions, you now have the capacity to focus yourself in your lovemaking toward achieving an orgasm that doesn't rely on just one trigger site, but on a multiple of trigger sites that culminate in super sexual orgasm. For that is, in essence, what makes super sexual orgasm stand head and shoulders above all other sexual sensations for a woman. With SSO, you get a multitude of orgasmic sensations happening simultaneously. From the stimulation of the cul-de-sac, you get the deep sensation of a vaginal orgasm. It's almost like an orgasm within an orgasm, in fact. With the relaxing and spasming of your PC muscle around your lover's penis, you are experiencing what you may have traditionally felt to be your orgasm. And then with the excitement of your G-spot and clitoris, all your sensual bases are magnificently covered.

So truly, then, your super sexual orgasm is an all-encompassing sexual experience, the likes of which you can produce for yourself and for your lover again and again and again.

In Part II of this book, we will continue to enhance the SSO experience through the use of intimate bonding techniques and other special exercises. You will rise to even greater heights of pleasure as you add levels of depth and meaning to the SSO experience. But you have completed the basics and done a fine job, and right now you deserve a rest.

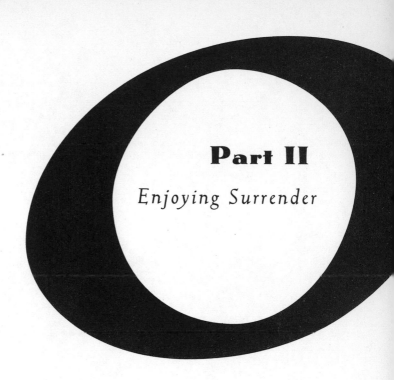

Part II

Enjoying Surrender

5

Bonding

*i*t is my deeply held belief, and my experience as well, that the greatest pleasure in learning how to experience super sexual orgasm is being able to share that thrill again and again with a loving partner. But this pleasure is, in many ways, also a necessity. To consistently achieve breathtaking SSOs, most women need far more than their partner's cooperation. They need a consistent sense of his caring and his trust.

But your partner has needs also. Your partner needs caring. Your partner needs to feel trust. And your partner needs to have information. In my clinical work, I often hear men complain that they can feel very left out of lovemaking. Female sexuality can seem terribly complex and intimidating at times, even to a very savvy partner. And the power of SSO can be particularly intimidating.

You don't want this to be a roadblock on the path to the pleasures of super sexual orgasm. When there is a man in your life who cares about your pleasure, he deserves to be an important part of your experience. And the closer the connection between the two of you, the more gratifying that experience will be. Now, more than ever, you have so much to share. You have already experienced your first super sexual orgasm, and that is an extraordinary prize. But in this chapter, I want you to go for the gold: increased personal sexual fulfillment *and* increased intimacy with another human being. Isn't it worth taking a little time right now to fortify your loving connection, and pave a path for a future of intimate sharing?

This chapter, written for you and your partner to read together, is all about connection. It will help both you and your partner understand the real value of his participation while demystifying your pursuit of the ultimate orgasm. And it will also offer him a number of techniques that greatly enhance the sensuality of his experience, while adding to the magic of yours.

Given the foundation that your partner is a decent and sensitive person, you can look forward with joy to the exercises in this chapter and the chapter that follows. I've found in all my therapeutic experience there is nothing that brings a couple to sexual rapture more than learning about each other's bodies together. A wellspring of totally consuming orgasms comes from each person in a loving partnership gaining an understanding of his or her own and his or her partner's sexual and sensual needs. The techniques I will outline for you are crafted specifically to help you and your partner meet these powerfully intertwined needs. By figuratively and sometimes literally guiding your partner's hand to a greater knowledge of the pleasures of your body, the two of you will form a powerful emotional and spiritual as well as physical bond. The lovemaking that blossoms from this cannot help but be profoundly ecstatic.

A TIME FOR *US*

As I said before, this chapter has been written for you and your partner to read together, and I hope that you do just that. Present this not as a demand but as an option, as an avenue of augmented sexual exploration for the two of you. I've even known some couples to turn the reading of some of my previous books into part of their lovemaking, the ultimate compliment I could ever receive.

In any event, whether or not this chapter becomes a bedtime story for the two of you, there is one thing you must both agree on at the start. This seems pretty basic, but it eludes a lot of people: You must mutually agree to schedule convenient times to do these exercises together. At these times, you should be ready to fully engage in the process—mentally, physically, and emotionally.

If at a given time, you are not available on those three

levels or perhaps your partner is not, be honest about it with each other and reschedule. Or perhaps you can do whatever few things need to be done to settle the situation and move on into the exercises. But be realistic. There are always going to be reasons you or your lover could look to for rescheduling to a better time almost every time. As they say, it's always something. So don't get caught up in a merry-go-round of finding the "perfect" time. A good time is good enough.

One more thing. Make sure that the place you do the exercises—and it does not have to be your bedroom necessarily—is comfortable, totally private, and free of distractions. If you want to try out a number of different places to see what works best, go ahead. But, if possible, just so you can establish some kind of supportive, consistent environmental rhythm, try to narrow your location down to one in particular as soon as possible.

SPOKEN WORD

A critical element to conclude each of the following exercises with is *talking*—talking about what you have done and how this has made you feel. You don't have to give a Ph.D. defense about your experience. A few words may suffice. You'll see. Most important, speak from the heart as you talk and be honest about yourself.

When you listen, do just that. Don't interrupt. Don't think about what you are going to say in response. Let the information in. You may disagree. Okay. Nothing wrong with that. Just don't turn this into a sporting event with everything being about winning and losing. Intimacy is never about winning and losing; it's about communicating and growing.

Feel free to ask each other questions, such as: How did you feel during this and that part of the exercise? Was there a portion that was more enjoyable, scary, weird? How was your concentration? Did you lose it? When? And how did you get it back? These and other questions can be asked again and again with greatly revealing results for the two of you.

And please note, if you decide to make any changes based on the information you receive, they should be changes you will try, not changes you will necessarily make forever. Each experience of the exercises keeps the dynamism of the interplay going. The pleasure patterns you will create together will be infinite if you just allow yourselves to be.

TO BOND, WITH LOVE

The exercises you are going to work on with your partner in this chapter are what I consider to be the essentials, the primary colors so to speak, of any relationship. I like to call these "bonding techniques." You may find them sexy, even a total turn-on, but that is not their primary focus. The goal here is to enhance feelings of closeness, intimacy, trust, and acceptance. You will be holding, cuddling, hugging, and playing. You will become relaxed with each other, attuned in such a fine way that your breathing and heartbeats may even fall into rhythm together. Actions speak louder than words. And so you may find that even if you have told your partner "I love you" many, many times, this love deepens incredibly after doing these exercises. This is also why I suggest you do one or more of these exercises for at least ten minutes a day, every day of your relationship lives.

EMBRACEABLE YOU

In the first bonding exercise, you are going to practice "spoon breathing." Here's how it's done.

Lie together, nude or clothed, on a comfortable surface with one person's back snuggled up against the other person's front. The person who is in back places a hand on the stomach of the person in front. Lie perfectly still and try not to talk or wiggle. Pay attention alternately to your breathing and your partner's breathing. Take three to four deep breaths and exhale forcefully. This should start to slow your breathing down. Do this several times. If you notice you are starting to breathe quickly again, take these deep breaths. Make sure your muscles are relaxed. Go through your body muscle by muscle and check each one for tension. Release, release, release. Let the warmth and the closeness you are feeling to your lover wash over you and bathe you in peace and tranquility.

You may notice that after a few minutes of spoon breathing you actually feel lighter throughout your whole body, and that your partner feels lighter too. A lot of couples like to fall asleep in this position. I also recommend spoon breathing when one or the other of you is headachy or feeling out of sorts. Some couples even do this when one of them is sick. There is no hard clinical proof for this, but many people in my practice have told me it helps their ill partner heal more quickly. I can understand why.

THE EYE OF THE BEHOLDER

Eye gazing is a bonding exercise that many couples find even more intimate than spoon breathing. See for yourself.

Again, lie on a comfortable surface and face each other. It is your choice whether to be naked or clothed. Wrap your arms comfortably around each other and gaze into each other's eyes for several minutes without talking, making sounds, or pantomiming.

Couples have reported to me that such intense feelings of closeness well up for them during this exercise that one or the other or both have started trembling. Some have even started crying as their hearts open up without interference to each other. Even if your reaction is not as strong, such prolonged eye contact rejuvenates the senses and the soul. It builds love and promotes acceptance. How wonderful to have your precious partner in your arms.

LAP OF LUXURY

Lap dancing may be all the rage right now, but it has nothing on this next beautiful exercise. I'm sure you'll both agree.

Sit with your back against a wall or other vertical surface. Your partner lies down with his head in your lap in such a way that he feels comfortable. Tenderly wrap your arms around him, sometimes soothing his forehead with gentle loving strokes. Share this embrace and feel each other's warmth. Breathe. Feel your hearts beat. Then switch places and repeat the exercise.

FULL-BODY CONTACT

Have you ever wanted to feel as much of your partner as you could all at one time? Well, now you can, or close to it, with the following technique.

Lie on your back on a comfortable surface and have your partner slowly lower himself on top of you, nose to nose. He should gradually, sensuously allow his full weight to be supported by you on the bottom. Stay this way for at least five minutes, silent and attentive to each other. Sense your lover at every point of contact. Do not talk or make any active efforts to move.

You can do this exercise either clothed or in the buff. Surprisingly, it does not seem to make much difference if one person is much heavier or taller than another. No one is overwhelmed because the mass of body spread out against body finds its own equilibrium. Adjust your head to a place of greatest comfort. Some people like having their faces nose to nose while others like to lie cheek to cheek.

When you are done, switch places and repeat the exercise.

Everyone needs a little nurturing in his or her life. Yet too often we forget to ask our lover what he or she would like—and if we are not asked, we forget to ask for ourselves as well. We go around assuming and hoping that our dearest can see into our mind and heart and must know when we want what we want. And if we don't get that kind of clairvoyance, well then, we get quite out of sorts about it.

But being in a relationship does not suddenly impart to you or your lover the omnipotent ability to know what the other person wants without him or her saying it. Sometimes you can guess right or pick up on subtle clues. But the best policy is to ask for what you want in a loving way. And if you ask for any of these loving bonding exercises, I guarantee you are going to cherish some incredible moments of gentle, soothing support that all of us long for and deserve on a daily basis.

A CARESS IS SOMETHING TO SHARE

In Part I of this book, you learned about the sensate focus caress, and had a number of opportunities to practice a basic full-body caress and a very intimate genital caress. But this is just the tip of the sensate focus iceberg. And right now, it's time to move on to another level of partner bonding by broadening your repertoire of sensate focus caresses.

When you do any of the following partner sensate focus caresses, remember that one of you will be taking the *active* role and one of you will be taking the *passive* role. You will always switch roles halfway through each exercise, so it doesn't matter who goes first.

Alternating active and passive roles encourages important aspects of wholeness and balance in a relationship. Consciously or unconsciously, as a relationship progresses, each partner typically moves into a set of defined activities that becomes a role. These activities may be emotionally or task-oriented. They are often very low-key and subtle things. For instance, if you both shower together, perhaps one of you typically washes the other first. Or, here's a familiar scenario: One of you always picks up take-out food on the way home when you are not going to cook. Not a big deal? Maybe. But you would be surprised how many couples in a relationship crisis have been brought to that point in no small measure because patterns have entrenched and accumulated till the weight and intractability of it all has broken into the foundation of commitment.

Sensate focus exercises give both of you the opportunity to get outside your usual roles and routines. Being passive and active alternately takes away established limits on communication and requires you to both branch out and explore your entire individual self and selves in altogether new ways. So many couples I know have told me the sensate focus exercises have functioned as a tonic and elixir, filling their emotional and spiritual lives with honor, integrity, and joyous equality. Plus, I might add, the exercises feel great and are a whole lot of fun.

A few more thoughts before we get into the exercises: Sensate focus is for your pleasure. Touching your partner while concentrating on what feels good to you may seem selfish, but it is in fact good for the both of you. Mutuality is promoted because you will both focus on a shared activity at the same time. You will both be consummately together in the moment. When you are the active partner, add to your focus on touch a focus on creating a positive, healing energy directed toward your passive mate. And when you are the passive partner, just relax and enjoy the caress, unless of course something bothers you and you want your partner to stop.

As I've mentioned earlier, if during these exercises disquieting emotional material comes up for you or you feel in any way physically compromised, whether you understand why or not, immediately cease the activity. Consider discussing this immediately with a therapist or other health professional.

FACE VALUE

You and your partner want to start the process of being intimately absorbed and involved with each other through a sensate focus face caress. As with all the exercises to follow, I suggest allowing a one-hour minimum of time together. You may feel like moving into lovemaking afterward but remember, this is not a requirement.

The sensate focus touching time is enough in and of itself. You may want to use a skin lotion as a part of this exercise, but it is not mandatory. I suggest removing watches, rings, and bracelets so that your hands and arms are soft everywhere to the touch.

As the active partner, sit with your back against a vertical surface (a wall, a headboard, etc.) with a pillow on your lap. Your partner should lie between your legs, face up, head on the pillow. It is important to have your partner's face within easy reach. If using lotion, begin to caress your partner's face, stroking everything from the top of the head to the base of his neck. At all times move slowly, sensuously, and lightly. If you remember to focus on feeling the skin, not the muscles underneath the skin, the pressure you apply will stay just right.

Move one or both hands across your partner's forehead and down the cheeks in a circular motion. Take deep belly breaths as you do so. Caress your lover's chin and dwell on every centimeter of skin on his neck and ears. The nose and eyelids are also places of extremely delicious sensory pleasure. Find all the spots that turn you on. After fifteen minutes, switch roles.

THE LONG, GOOD BACK CARESS

In this next exercise, the sensate focus back caress, you will caress the entire back side of your partner's body, from neck to feet. As always, conduct the session in a comfortable environment. I also suggest warming up for the exercise with five minutes of spoon breathing.

To start, have your partner lie facedown. He can keep his arms at his sides or underneath his head. Lie alongside him, maintaining as much body contact as possible during the exercise. Stroke your partner's back sensuously and slowly with a hand. You can start anywhere, but the first time through, start at the neck. Run any portion of your hand—fingers, knuckles, palm, heel of the palm—over the shoulder blades and then down the spine. Drift your hand over your lover's buttocks and legs.

Think of your partner's body as a sensory playground and touch anything that feels good to you. Explore and enjoy the sensuality of your partner's back with different strokes. This is not a massage, though, so keep your touch light. Stay attuned to differences in temperature, texture, and shape. Try caressing with your eyes closed and see how that affects how you sense what you are touching. Use lotion or baby power if you like, especially if your hands tend to perspire. If you sense your partner's body tensing during the caress, lightly press down on the tensing area as a signal to your partner to relax.

If you have trouble focusing, consciously slow your caressing motion down to half the speed it was before. If thoughts about what your partner is feeling intrude, bring your mind back to the exact point of contact between your skin and your partner's skin. The only thing you need to think of in relation to your partner is how he feels to you. Remember that each stroke of your hand sends healing goodwill toward your loved one without saying any words or making any sounds.

After about twenty minutes, do five minutes of spoon breathing before changing roles. At the end of the hour, spoon *breathe together again before either getting dressed or moving on further with your lovemaking.*

This next exercise is a sensual variation on the back caress you just learned.

Begin your sensate focus back caress, but this time instead of caressing with your hands, use some other part of your upper body, such as your hair, face, or breasts, or try using your feet. Each will engender in you a unique and extraordinary range of sensory experiences.

If you become sexually aroused during this back caress enjoy it, but bring your mind back to experiencing the point of contact between you and your partner. There can be time for lovemaking later on.

After twenty minutes, spoon breathe and change roles. When you are the passive partner, soak up the sensations like a sponge. Breathe evenly, deeply, and regularly. Relax your muscles. Keep your mind on the precise point of contact where your partner strokes you. Try not to move. Accept the stimulation you receive and only speak up if something feels uncomfortable or inappropriate. Spoon breathe again at the conclusion of the exercise.

UP FRONT AND PERSONAL

In this exercise you and your lover get to lavish attention on the other side of the body. Your caress will include the genital area, but not in any detailed way. There will be no penetration of the vagina, for instance, just stroking the outside of it, because this is a sensual exercise not a sexual one. Make all your preparations for yourselves and your environment before you begin, and, as before, allow the same amount of quiet time.

Begin with five minutes of spoon breathing. After your spoon breathing the passive partner lies on his back, and you, the active partner, lie next to him. Maintain as much full-body contact as possible. You can try resting your hand or cheek against your lover's chest to listen for a heartbeat for a few minutes. Then begin stroking your mate, ever so slowly, starting with his face, neck, shoulders, and arms. Move down to the chest, stomach, abdomen, and genitals, and farther to the thighs, calves, feet, and toes.

After a full experience using your hands, start again from the beginning. This time, however, caress with your face, hair, or breasts. Close your eyes and move extra slowly. Release into the intense energy of the moment. Finish up by listening to your partner's heartbeat. Spoon breathe and then switch roles. Spoon breathe again at the conclusion of the exercise.

The conversation you have relating to how this particular caress affected you both should be quite amazing. It is so very intimate, and for many, transcendent.

TWO INFORMED ADULTS ON A MATTRESS

This next exercise can be very erotic, but more important, it is educational. You would be amazed at how many men and women say they know all about a woman's genital anatomy but give me physical details that are closer to describing a chicken than a human being. I'd like to say they were taught by nuns, as I was, but I know that's not always the case. I think this lack of knowledge is linked to the shame and embarrassment that society manages to subtly and not-so-subtly convey to us about our genitals (even though other segments of society, like advertising, use our sexuality to blatantly titillate us, but I don't want to get into a whole sociological analysis here). What I want is for you to spend some intimate time going over your genital terrain with your lover. So get comfortable (maybe begin with a body caress or some of the other bonding exercises in this chapter), get a flashlight, then get to the exercise.

The goal of this exercise is to help your partner get more comfortable with and wise about your body. So remove all of your clothing and invite him to learn.

The structures you want to make sure you're both clear on to start are the outer lips and inner lips of your vagina, the hood that covers the clitoris, and then the clitoris itself. This isn't a budget tour so take your time. You don't have to look like you're doing an autopsy either—smile or giggle if you want. Breathe. Lighten up.

Have your lover insert a finger sensuously into your vagina and feel the PC muscle. Tighten and release it. Have him curve his finger up, pointing toward the mound to identify the G-spot—it has a rough feel.

Now have your lover take a lubricated dildo and insert it gently into you. Tighten the PC muscle and let him see how it holds. Release the muscle and do the vaginal breathing that allows for the opening of the cul-de-sac. Let him see how the dildo goes in that extra space and how the cul-de-sac closes in on it. Tug lightly on the dildo and let him see how it holds in place.

If you get excited doing this, even to the point of orgasm, enjoy your journey. But try to keep making it educational for him. Make every effort to point out the color and texture changes that occur as you become aroused. Pinks become reds, muscles tighten and spasm, tissues swell, and areas lubricate. It is all a beautiful, natural part of the sensual dance.

MORE READY THAN EVER

Congratulations. You have now completed all of the bonding techniques—techniques which are certain to enhance all aspects of your lovemaking. Frankly, I feel that the exercises you have just completed are the most difficult exercises in this book; difficult because they involve such intimate emotional risks. But you've succeeded. And you should be very proud of yourself and proud of the relationship you have just strengthened. Now you can move on, taking your partner with you for the rest of your wild SSO ride. When you need him most, he will be there for you, and his strength will give you strength.

But be prepared, also, for a few surprises. The new, greater strength of your bond may bring forth a very unexpected additional payoff into your lovemaking experience: transcendence. I think I better explain . . .

Perhaps you've read or heard, particularly in Eastern cultures, about how some kinds of lovemaking can lead to spiritual, ecstatic, almost altered states in which you feel connected to something larger than yourself. Well, this is exactly the kind of sensation many women describe experiencing with their partners once they incorporate these bonding techniques into their SSO lovemaking.

Now, I am not very religious and I don't consider myself especially spiritual. In fact, my friends would probably say I'm one of the most skeptical, "show me exactly how that works and why" people around. And yet after I started experimenting personally with SSOs, I too would have to say my lovemaking sessions took on a quality of transcendence to another realm. Every woman's experiences are personalized, but here, as examples, are my own observations.

During SSO sex everything looks clearer, sharper, and brighter. Sometimes I have seen colored flashing lights, sometimes I have heard faint, ethereal music, sometimes I have felt as if I was levitated off the bed. And one time, in a giant illumination of brightness, I felt I could actually see the union of my partner's and my souls. The state of pleasure was so intense at times that I felt a serene blissfulness not unlike what Buddhism describes as a state of being free from desire. So transported was I by the cosmic intensity of this feeling, it was like I was floating, wondering if I was before, in, or after orgasm.

None of this, by the way, was anything I willed or consciously made happen. Yes, the ecstatic experiences came out of my own freed sexuality to be sure. But when they happened, they happened *to* me, taking their own natural course.

EAST MEETS WEST

Let's take a big step back for a second. Even from a purely physiological point of view, cul-de-sac penetration is a very intense experience. Could all that I have just described spring from the physiological reality that one is panting so much as to hyperventilate, and that there is an accompanying massive release of endorphins? To be sure, all this is going on. All I can say, however, is once you have yourself felt the transformation that SSO brings, you will be hard-pressed to write it off as just a biological phenomenon. The results of an SSO sexual union point toward an ecstatic connection with a higher power, whether for you that power is God, pure light, goddesses and spirit guides, or Nature.

Even if you appreciate the following information on a purely intellectual as opposed to a spiritual level, I think you will find it worth considering that in Eastern traditions, the universe is regarded as being created by the union of the male and female—pure consciousness (Shiva/male) and pure energy (Shakti/female). The universe is sustained on a macrocosmic level by this interplay of male and female. On the microcosmic human sexuality level, I believe the same need for interplay and balance is required. In order to explore the furthest reaches of lovemaking potential, a woman needs to explore her male side by learning to have very explosive orgasms. A man needs to explore his female side by containing his orgasmic energy and controlling his ejaculation while still having orgasms.

The way to go beyond arousal, beyond mutuality, beyond intimacy, and to ecstasy requires that a woman find a partner who worships her body, especially the sacred space of her vagina. For a man, that quest for ecstasy requires that he find a mate who lovingly accepts his penis, and to whom he can open his heart. The ultimate union will see a couple speaking to each other and respecting each other through their genitals. Such communication will only happen when both parties bring their full sexuality to the union and when both are completely present in every loving moment of embrace.

6
Icing

s with all good journeys, what looks like the end of the road is, when more closely examined, actually the beginning of a new adventure. While super sexual orgasm, in certain ways, constitutes the pinnacle of sexual sensation you can feel during penetration, it is far from being the only breathtaking height you can experience.

To experience the power of super sexual orgasm it was necessary to practice many exercises and master certain techniques. But these same exercises and techniques have a number of additional, equally exciting applications for any woman who is interested in further expanding her sensual repertoire and surrendering even further to her own sexual power.

To me, SSO is the cake. But now it is time for the icing. And there is, in fact, so much icing, so much more sensuality that you can bring to your SSO lovemaking, that I have felt hard-pressed to decide which of my favorite tips for added intimacy to include in these pages. I love cake. But my favorite part is the icing. Do you feel the same way? Then survey the opportunities I am about to reveal to you, and sample from them till you find out what suits your taste.

But a word to the wise before we get started: Do not think in terms of having to master all of these techniques now, or even ever. This is not the place for feeling that you have to do everything everyone does, and do it better than they do. Lighten up, get into a mind-set of wanting to have fun, dust off your sense of humor, and dive into the sea of sensual possibilities. Follow your instincts to arrive at a sexual repertoire that works for you. Not that the repertoire you arrive at will be static, either. What you like will change for all kinds of reasons: different moods, different partners, different time of the year, different locations—just to name a few reasons. You may have enough of something you thought you would love doing forever. And then, just as suddenly, you may become intrigued with something that up until that moment never held any charm for you.

This ever-changing nature of what appeals to your

sense of sexuality is what makes the lovemaking experience so profoundly magical. And it's the way of the sexual world.

SOUNDS LIKE SEXUAL SPIRIT

In the majority of the exercises in this book, we focused
on the power of touch as a means of connecting with
your sensual self. Now it's time to bring the element of
sound into the sexual equation. Notice I didn't say talking. Because what we are going to explore in the next few
exercises includes talking, but encompasses an even
wider range of vocalization.

What is an orgasm? We've already talked about this a
lot. And I'm sure that by now, you have your own
thoughts and feelings to add to the discussion. Maybe
even a little poetry. But the bottom line is this: An
orgasm is a release—an intense, concentrated release of
energy—and the greater the release, the stronger the
orgasm.

It follows logically, then, that any way you can add to
such a release will heighten the experience of orgasm and
all that leads up to it. Little os become big Os, and super
sexual orgasms become super-duper sexual orgasms. When
you intensify your sexual experiences by adding in the
vocalization factor, you will intensify your feelings, escalate
your energy release, and amplify your SSO ecstasy multi-
fold.

You've probably experienced this phenomenon in the
nonsexual arena many times and just never even paid

attention to what you were doing. But take a moment to reflect on what I'm saying now. Here, let me give you some examples to think about. For instance, if you've ever ridden on a roller coaster, didn't you feel your level of thrill increase when you screamed as you soared and plummeted at breakneck speed? If you've ever watched a baseball game at a stadium, didn't you join in with the crowd by cheering, yelling, or chanting when your team scored a run—and didn't this excite you even more? When you make dinner or hang around in the kitchen sampling what your partner has made, don't you either say something or make some sound of approval when you taste something especially good—and doesn't what you are tasting seem to taste better yet? I'm sure now that I've got you thinking along these lines, you can come up with many more of your own examples where sound enhanced an experience.

The point is, sex is no different from any of these other examples you can think up from your own life. Simply put, the most magnificent sex is not silent. Sure, you can have some delicious silent encounters. But all my years of work as a sexual surrogate and then as a sex therapist have led me to the conclusion that vocalization—whatever that means for each individual—is absolutely essential to experiencing your most complete orgasm. And that includes the super sexual orgasm. If you give your lovemaking all you've got—the full range of sounds and words you have inside of you—then you will discover that your sex life has a lot more than you ever thought or previously experienced to give back to you.

BREAKING THE SOUND BARRIER

But wait. Are you just a little uncomfortable about this vocalization thing? After all, if you speak up, well then, won't you be heard? And don't many of us have an early ingrained training of being "good little girls" who were as silent, polite, ladylike, and compliant as possible in all aspects of our lives? And when we did speak up, weren't we expected to say something nice and soothing or at least agreeable? And aren't the sounds that might come out of your mouth during sex—if you were to truly let go—likely to be raw, animalistic, unbridled, guttural, volcanically panting, maybe even stridently dirty? Does this potential inside of you frighten you and make you want to wear a baffle on your head?

It does to many, many women. Which is why, before we do finally get down to it, I want to explore with you what apprehensions you might be feeling at this moment, especially if making sounds during sex is something you are not accustomed to. I firmly believe that the fear of releasing the sounds we have inside of us—be they words, cries, grunts, shrieks, fragments of words, or sentences (or even an incomprehensible melange of all of this)—during any activity, but especially during sex, is a *learned* behavior.

I mentioned previously how for many of us, our upbringing to be "good little girls" often resulted in us being stifled from expressing what we really felt like saying. And then after the stiflers were no longer there in our lives to continue such stifling, we took on their role and often muffled ourselves into silence better than anyone ever had before. Good girls do everything well, you see, even when it ends up hurting themselves.

In my house growing up, speaking about sex—and certainly hearing the sounds of lovemaking—was scrupulously avoided. You would have thought my mother was involved in a series of virgin births, so carefully was any iota of sexuality excised from our family environment. If you came from this kind of household, or even one that was not that extreme but where there was still a level of unease around the facts of sexuality, you may have started feeling that sexual activity and its related sounds were dirty, or scary, or weird, or worse yet, something to be minimized.

Even if you came from a family environment where sex was not the big taboo, you may have developed a hesitation around or pattern of avoidance of making sounds during lovemaking because of certain life situations. Situations like these, for example: When you were in college, you were conscious that a roommate might be listening or that you might wake up the whole dorm if you really let it rip during your orgasm; in adult life, you didn't want to have the entire condo complex aware of when you were getting "lucky"; or even now that you have your own home, you feel constrained about waking up the kids or making any kind of noise that would disturb the dog and make her start howling.

And even if you managed to come from a well-balanced family in which sex received the "don't ask, don't tell" treatment, and even if you didn't have any of the living situations I just outlined, you still might not be giving full rein to your sexual voice because it would reveal too much about you. Yes, because letting out what you have inside of you spontaneously during sex does say a lot about you in that you are opening yourself to your deepest, most personal core—and that's scary for any one of us. It's asking us to trust ourselves, and our partners—a lot to let that core be revealed and not derided or belittled or smirked at or smiled at in any way. This is tough stuff to accomplish, even for the best balanced, most emotionally even keel among us.

What I'm saying here is, I know that asking you to become vocal during lovemaking requires a lot from you, emotionally, spiritually, and physically. It has been tough for almost all of us at one point or another in our lives. So please, as I've said in all the chapters before this, go at your own pace. Don't do what doesn't feel comfortable to you. Take "small bites," not big mouthfuls. Chew everything well and think about what you're absorbing. And just make sure that your partner clearly understands he will need to share with you, now more than ever before, all his caring, love, patience, and sincere, undivided attention to help you sustain an environment where it is safe to be heard in this world.

THE ART OF NOISE

Let's loosen up your vocal cords with a simple exercise before you start adding a soundtrack to your lovemaking sessions. Some people feel it helps to play music as a background to mask the sounds they will make during this exercise. And other people like going to a location like a park or an empty beach where they can make as much noise as they want without disturbing anyone. It's basically up to you. Just make sure that you choose a location where you are comfortable making as much noise as you can possibly make.

Take a book with dialogue (you can also take a poem or a screenplay or a play if you like) and start reading it aloud. Begin in a normal tone of voice. Give the words the inflection you feel they should have and don't worry about whether an acting coach would approve. After a few lines, start to increase the volume at which you are reading, and as you do so experiment with adding intonations that have nothing to do with the words or the meaning and in fact make no sense at all. Then, as you are continuing to read out loud in an elevated tone of voice, start adding in random grunts, guffaws, giggles, screams, and any other sounds you can come up with. Hum even. In the middle of it all, drop your voice to a whisper and then in the next second explode all the way out to your loudest voice.

Put aside the text and continue to make only loud sounds, dropping out the talking altogether. If moving around helps you do this, feel free to sway, dance, hop, glide, fox trot—whatever literally moves you. And remember to take deep, enriching breaths and remain relaxed throughout your body, most especially in your vocal cords.

Keep these noise sessions to about five minutes each to start with so that you will not overdo things and get laryngitis. Give yourself at least a week to start feeling comfortable with the high-end range of what your voice can emit.

When you get comfortable and confident in your voice noise-making it is as if a whole other dimension has been added to your life and your love life. I've had some clients tell me that this exercise alone was the pivotal one for them, the moment that released them from years of living their life in the silent shadows. You may have the same experience or this exercise might just be the beginning of the releasing process for you. The important thing is not to have any set expectations. Just enjoy the exercise for what it does for you. And then get ready to move on to your next vocal assignment.

GO YELL IT ON THE MOUNTAIN

In this exercise, which is a partner exercise, you and your partner are going to make the wildest range of noises you can come up with. As in the previous exercise, you can choose to stay indoors or outside. The only requirement is that you don't put any limits on the levels of sound you will both make. Also, do not make any physical contact during the course of the exercise. But again, if you feel the inclination to make any kind of movements during the process that only involve yourself, then definitely go ahead.

Begin by making sure you are relaxed throughout your body. Take deep easy breaths. Increase the pace of your breathing and make your breaths audible. Now start to make any kind of nonverbal noise that comes into your mind. Try not to think too much about what you are doing, but let go in a stream of noise consciousness. Mimic your partner if you like or make the sound he is making in a slightly different way. Keep increasing the sound level of your voices as you laugh, gurgle, roar, whinny, burp, and snore, to name a few noises you can make. Look at each other as you reach the top of your decibel range and see if you can project your voice as if into each other's being. Keep that high-energy bond going. And then, if you can manage to do this simultaneously, suddenly let your voices drop. Keep breathing audibly. Move the air smoothly in and out of your lungs. Check your body out muscle by muscle to make sure you are relaxed and then, while continuing to stare into each other's eyes, take the time to let your breathing settle down to a normal rate.

In this playacting technique, each partner takes turns making the sounds he or she thinks a wildly orgasmic person would make. This is your opportunity go way over the top with your vocalization. Dramatization and bad dinner theater here you come. Send out your sounds so that people on the other side of the world can wake up and hear you. We're talking along the lines of Meg Ryan's bravura orgasm imitation performance in When Harry Met Sally. Give Meg a run for her money and put on a knock-down-drag-out orgasm show for yourself and your partner.

Now here's the wacky part. Switch roles. Yes, now you get to imitate the ultimate orgasm you think a man would express. And your partner will then get a chance at trying his voice at being a woman in the throes of an SSO. This is not about changing the pitch of your voice. Actually try to generate the sounds you have heard your mate express, but add into it your own creativity and vital force. Give your performance the intensity of a rocket launch and see if you can make the sparks fly!

BASIC INSTINCTS

This next exercise is one of the most popular vocalization techniques I've developed for my clients over the years. When I ask why it has such appeal, I most often get the answer that it is a lot of fun and connects with something very basic inside of everyone. Here's how it goes.

One of you will be the active partner and the other the passive partner. At the end of the exercise you will switch roles. The active partner is going to sensually caress the passive partner, all the while making sounds like our ancestors the cavepeople might have made. So imagine yourself in a loincloth and go to it! Bellow, purr, yelp, grunt—whatever suits your fancy. Just make sure not to talk. Don't utter even one word. Channel everything you are feeling into sounds.

A lot of people tell me they feel really motivated to continue into lovemaking and orgasm after this exercise. I feel this is naturally the case because the playacting of being cavepeople really helps us get away from all the mental barriers we often bring into our sexual encounters: Am I doing this right? How do I look? How do I sound? If our ancestors had these kind of hang-ups they

sure didn't leave any mention of it on their wall paint-
ings. So the next time you start feeling superior to Cro-
Magnon woman, be a little kinder in your outlook. With
respect to how she experienced her sex life at least, she
most likely had quite a lot on the ball.

TALK IS CHEAP . . . AND SEXY

From here on out, the exercises we will be exploring will
not only include sounds, but will also include words. It's
not that these verbal techniques are more advanced or
any more special than the nonverbal exercises we did
before. They all have a value and, as I said in the beginning of this chapter, different people will find different
exercises to be more or less of a turn-on. So what I advise
you to do is try your hand, and mouth, and whatever
other part of your body you find appealing, at the exercises and see what creates the best animal magnetism
between you and your partner.

*Have your partner lie facedown, fully clothed, on a comfortable
surface. You will sit down next to him and quietly study what
you can see exposed of his body—starting for instance with his
hair, head, and neck. First, express through sounds how
looking at these parts of his body makes you feel. Then, after
you have taken your time doing this, put this feeling into
words. Remember, you're not going for a description of your
lover—you're trying to vocalize the effect his presence is having
on you. Don't be modest, polite, or discreet. Go for the sensual,
sexual, animalistic jugular. Use your voice in a sexual way,*

exciting your lover, but most of all truly expressing your innermost desires.

Move on to removing your lover's shirt. Take in these new, alluring vistas of skin, curves, and muscle, and sound out just how excited this vision is making you. Then let your words out of you like a heated, heady lava of passion and lust. In this manner, strip your lover bit by bit, all the while appreciating him first in sound, then in word. When you have experienced him from head to toe, have him turn over onto his back and start the whole process over again, moving from his top to his toes. And when you are all done, exchange places and feel how erotic it can be to have someone sinuously appreciate you in a caress of sound.

HAND TO MOUTH

What you have been caressing only with your eyes and voice, you will now, in this next exercise, actually get to feel with your partner at the same time.

This exercise is similar to the previous one, except that you are going to touch your lover with whatever part of your body you are moved to use: tongue, ear lobe, big toe, buttocks—the choice is up to you. And as you are doing so, you are going to express through sound and word what this touch is making you feel like.

Again, don't censor what rises into your mind. Just feel it and translate it as fast as possible. If you find it easier to make sounds than words, that is fine, as long as you are expressing what is welling up inside of you. Some people are just naturally more communicative in sound rather than in words. When you move from a naturally relaxed place, you will find the vocal expression in this exercise that is right for who you are.

Remember to switch places after finishing the sensual and vocal exploration of your partner. Relax, breathe deeply, and get ready for a heady experience. There's nothing like being appreciated in such an intimate way by your lover.

CLAIRE'S KNEE

This next exercise has got to be one of my favorites. Not because it is necessarily so sensual, although it can be, but really because I always have such a good time teaching it to clients or doing it myself. It brings out the humorous potential in all of us. And having a sense of playful fun when you are having sex is one of the best aphrodisiacs of all time.

Lie down next to your lover on a comfortable surface. You can both be clothed or nude, it is up to you. The idea here is to take various parts of your body and give them a voice. Let's say you take your elbow. If your elbow could speak, what would it say about your lover? Maybe it would say that it loves to maneuver around every curve in your partner's body, especially the curve between his genitals and upper thigh. Become that elbow and tell him. Now it's your partner's turn. He will pick a part of his body and have it say something about you. In this way you create a dialogue that can be as silly as all get out but can also be very revealing and tender.

Remember too that your body parts are free to express themselves in sounds as well as words. Have you ever heard a belly button moan? I have. And it's pretty darn sexy.

WORDS TO TOUCH BY

Remember your old friend, the genital caress? In this next exercise, you are going to bring it back for an encore performance, but with some interesting new modifications.

Begin your sensate focus genital caress. This time, after you have finished engaging in such an experience as the passive partner, you are going to tell your lover what you particularly liked. Be very specific. Don't just say, "That was really good" or "Wow, when you touched me that was terrific." Get into the detail: How his index finger sliding up and over your clitoris was incredible; how his tongue against your inner thigh was like a touch of sensuous fire. You get the idea. Present the information in a straightforward way, beginning your sentences with "I liked . . . ," "I enjoyed . . . ," or "I loved . . ." By making these kinds of statements, you learn to be clear, assertive, and confident when talking about sex in general and about what you want out of sex in particular.

When you make your "I" statements, be sincere. Don't think you have to massage your mate's ego. Just give him a direct communication about what he did that really turned you on. If there was one thing, that's okay. Just tell him that. If your partner does not understand exactly what you mean, restate your comment. Remember, as the passive partner, you need to

*stay out of your head and remain specifically in your body, as
we have explored before in the sensate focus exercises. However,
in contrast to the way you kept silent during the sensate focus
caresses in previous chapters, if you are moved to make any
kind of sound this time, go right ahead.*

The active partner in this exercise needs to remember
this: Do not interpret a comment about one kind of touch
as meaning that your other touches were not good or not
interesting. Your partner is simply telling you what
seemed to be particularly sensual at that given moment—
something that might not be at all sensual if you did the
same thing tomorrow. The point is, certain touches in certain moments are especially thrilling. And if you have
good communication during sex, you can always keep
tabs on what those points of excitement are.

One more critical element for the active partner to
note. Always keep in mind that you are touching your
partner for your own pleasure. She will tell you what
turns out to be gratifying for her, but do not be motivated by trying to please her. Sometimes this is difficult
to remember to do if your partner starts to moan or
grunt in an appreciative way during some of the touching. Naturally, you may want to dwell on that area and
that kind of touching since it seems to be getting such a
great response. But you have to maintain your own satisfaction focus.

And by the way, feel free to make any kind of noises
you like as well during the exercise. Maintain the mind-
set in which you are able to touch for your own pleasure,

even though you know that your partner is enjoying the sensations too. When you are able to achieve a balance between your pleasure and that of your partner, you have arrived at a place of mutuality—a state of beautifully balanced sexual satisfaction for both man and woman.

After you have finished conveying your feelings to your partner this first time, have your partner pleasure you again with a second genital caress. Your partner should try to do things differently this time. Once again, when he is done, let him know how it felt for you this time. When you have been caressed twice in this manner, switch roles so that you are the active one caressing your mate.

SEX ON DEMAND

It's time to ask for exactly what you need. And get it too. You've waited a long time, but now all the barriers have been removed and nothing remains but your desire.

Start by being the active partner. In this role, you will get to ask your mate to do anything you want him to do, short of something that he finds uncomfortable or unpleasant. If he does not do exactly what you want, using the direct method of communication you learned in the previous exercise, clarify what you are after. Feel free to enjoy, for as long as you want, whatever you have asked your partner to do. If you want to talk or make noises while you are being pleasured, let yourself go to it.

The passive partner's job is to do what is asked of him in a sensual, sensate focus manner while you are concentrating on your own pleasure. See if you can reach that state of mutuality in which you are doing a caress so it feels good to you, but you are aware that your partner is enjoying it too. Make sounds if you like, when your body stirs them up inside of you.

Both of you need to come from a place of centeredness, relaxation, and being in the present moment. Active partner: Don't be thinking of what you want your partner to be doing one minute from now or ten minutes from now. Passive partner: Don't anticipate what you might be expected to do next. And certainly don't worry about whether you are being sensual or sexual enough. Just do what you have been asked to do and make yourself feel good doing it.

Go ahead and lose track of time as you make the intimate connection with your lover's body. And when you have finished, and are feeling fully satisfied, be sure to switch roles.

STREAM OF SEX CONSCIOUSNESS

This next exercise is a terrific exercise to strengthen trust between lovers.

Begin by lying on your back and having your partner perform a genital caress on you. Instead of just making sounds or talking as you did in the previous exercise, I want you to let what comes out of your mouth be a stream of consciousness. Let it rip. Don't censor. Don't edit. Don't second-guess. Just loosen up and release whatever the touches of your partner bring out of you. This material may include emotions, fragmented statements, noises, and parts of words. It's all fine to share. You may even find that you start to cry.

The active partner should caress in a way that feels good to him. Strangely enough, this exercise works just fine if you don't get focused on what your partner is saying. Make your attention connection with the point of contact you have to your partner's body.

Switch roles after a while and do the exercise again.

This is a powerfully charged experience you are sharing with each other, so end the event with some bonding moments like spoon breathing, or whatever other technique gives you a strong level of comfort and support. You may feel like you want to make love afterward and if you have the desire, definitely act on it. Many couples, however, find they prefer to drift off to sleep in each other's arms after such a revealing encounter.

FANTASY ISLAND

If you thought the previous exercise was a trust builder, hold on to your hat. What you are going to learn now will really cement the core of caring you are creating between you and your lover. This exercise combines masturbation and fantasy, and there are actually two ways to do it. In both scenarios, the active partner will masturbate while recounting a fantasy. The choice is for the passive partner, who can either just listen or listen and masturbate as well.

You will both lie together on a comfortable surface. If you are the active partner, begin to masturbate, taking care to focus on your own arousal. Make whatever sounds you need in order to turn yourself on. Stimulate yourself in the way that you would if your lover were not there. Decide whether you will allow him to look at you—it is much more releasing, by the way, if you agree to let him observe. As you become more and more aroused, start to spin a fantasy. It can involve you and your lover, you and someone else, even your lover and someone else. Make it hot, sensuous, and erotic. Be lavish with detail that draws on all five of the senses.

The passive partner needs to remember that the only thing being recounted here is fantasy. It is not something that the active partner necessarily wants to do in real life. Accept your partner's sexual thoughts as they are. Relax as you listen and appreciate the openness that your partner feels toward you to be able to share something so profoundly personal.

After you as the active partner have climaxed, take a few minutes to do a bonding exercise, then switch roles and repeat the exercise.

ROMPING ROOM

Hopefully you have done all the exercises in these chapters with a sense of fun and adventure. Now, I'm sure some of you may have been a tad too serious at times so I want to speak especially to you right now. In the next few exercises, I absolutely, imperatively, demand—no, command—that you loosen up. Get downright goofy if you want to take it that far, but by all means play, play, play. The spontaneity of sex play is the most releasing, most rejuvenating, most refreshing, experience in the world. I am going to give you some examples of fun and games that have worked for many of my clients. But feel free to feel the spirit and make up some wild, unbridled games of your own.

Get your rubber duckies and jump into the tub! The sensuous shower is a whole-body caress that takes place while you are both showering together. You are going to enjoy your body and your lover's body along with the added excitement of the soothing water flow. And as an extra bargain, you get to be clean.

There are a number of ways to take your shower. Some couples just find it a hoot to be in the shower together. You can do any of your sensate focus caresses in turn or you can mutually caress each other. Use liquid soap or gel and caress any part of your lover's body that makes you feel good. If you become aroused, just enjoy the feelings and let them take you wherever they go. Some people like to have intercourse in the shower. (Just be careful because some types of soap irritate the vagina or the penis.)

You can also make this a bath-time experience. You may want to create a mood in your bathroom with incense, candles, music—maybe even sip a little wine in the tub. But remember, all those elements are extras. The real treat is cuddled up right next to you.

It's time for a sensual dinner. Prepare a number of foods that you feel are very special. It will help if they are also juicy, slightly goopy or messy. Think along the lines of fruits, melted cheeses, meat that can be pulled off the bone, custards, and whipped cream. Whatever drinks you decide to have, use elegant glassware to give your dinner a lovely quality. Have some flowers arranged and maybe some candles burning on a nearby table. Your food, however, will be spread out on a comfortable floor surface on an old sheet or tarp that will protect against any spillage.

Take off your clothes and prepare to observe the following ground rules: No feeding yourself, no talking, and no utensils.

Before you start feeding each other, do some bonding exercises and then some sensate focus caresses. Now begin feeding each other. Eat with the goal of feeling every sensation as the food passes from your lover's fingers to your lips and into your mouth. Put food on your body and offer it to your partner to lick or suck off. Kiss in between swallowing mouthfuls of food and drink.

Finish your sensually sumptuous evening by washing each other off slowly with warm wet towels or perhaps by taking a shower or bath together. And then? Well . . . the rest of the evening is up to you.

Designing tattoos on each other with washable—sometimes even edible—finger paints can be a wonderful way to spend an afternoon with your lover. Try this exercise in the bathtub or any part of the house that you have protected with some sheets or toweling. You may also want to try this outdoors. I've known some people to do this at nude beaches in California. (Where else?)

Be outlandish in your designs. Spell out racy words and draw erotic designs on each other. Use this game as a gateway into the more animalistic, primal aspect of your sexuality. Moan, growl, and lightly chew or suck on your lover as you *decorate. Put on some music with a great bass beat and parade around when you are done. Jungle love, here you come!*

THE FEELING IS MUTUAL

Mutual orgasm, which is sometimes also called simultaneous orgasm, is an amazing feeling. It refers to a couple having an orgasm at the same time during intercourse. A lot of people pooh-pooh this idea, and discourage others from trying it. Too much pressure, they say, and too little success. Granted, when you are not in control of your body mutual orgasm is more a product of luck than anything else and it should not be prioritized as a goal. But when you are in control, as you are now thanks to SSO, mutual orgasm is easily accomplished and absolutely fabulous.

In my way of thinking, mutual orgasm is much more than simply two orgasms happening at the same time. The most important aspect of it is that each lover enjoys the partner's orgasm as well as his or her own. Mutual orgasm is one of the most intimate experiences you can have with your lover. It is a celebration of all that is beautiful and sacred in the relationship you are building together. The union you create in that moment of mutual orgasm shoots right to the core of who you are as an individual and who you are as a couple as well.

In order to achieve such a mutually exalting experience, first start with some sensate focus caresses in order to relax and arouse each other. Then decide on a position to have intercourse, being sure to choose a position where you can look into each other's eyes. Bring your bodies together in your position of choice, knowing that whoever is on top will control the speed of the thrusting. Start slowly, enjoying every slight motion, every swirl and sway of your hips and thighs. As you roll through slow, sensuous thrusts, peak together through levels 6, 7, and 8.

Keep your motions shared and mutual as you thrust together and then slide apart. Relax, breathe, and focus on the sensations in your genitals. Women, think of your vagina as caressing your partner's penis. Men, think of your penis as licking the inside of your lover's vagina.

Peak up to level 9 and plateau there. With practice you will find that you can develop the ability to either hold back slightly at this highest level of arousal or accelerate your excitement to match that of your partner. As your partner spills over into orgasm, follow his plunge by taking a deep breath, relaxing every muscle, opening your eyes, and looking deep into his. Two climaxes in one long, loving moment.

SIMPLE PLEASURES ARE THE BEST

In all the discussions of sexual pleasure I have had with you, I haven't yet touched on the subject of kissing. Did I forget? No. Do I minimize it? Absolutely not. Then why am I only getting to it now? Because I like to save the best for last.

Kissing may be the most intimate, erotic experience you can share with your partner. Some of our most sensitive nerve endings are in our lips, so it is really no surprise that they feel and communicate with exquisite sensual precision. No wonder romance begins with a kiss.

With sensual kissing, you kiss as you would do any other sensate focus caress. You move slowly, you relax your lips, and you kiss for your own pleasure even though you are aware of your lover's sensitivities. As you stay in the here and now and focus on the kissing point of contact, notice the taste of your lover's mouth, the velvety feel, the rough feel, the warmth, the coolness, your partner's tongue, the motion and swirl of your partner's lips.

Gaze into your lover's eyes and feel your connection. You might graze your partner's lips or tongue with your teeth—not to hurt but to add some variety to the interaction. Kiss softly, seriously, slyly, slowly, sensuously. Don't think of where your kissing will lead. Just kiss.

Make time every day you are together to share your love through kissing. It may lead to lovemaking, but it is important to remember that kissing is a beautiful and fulfilling experience in and of itself. As long as you can share each other's kisses deep from the soul you will have a loving, secure place in each other's hearts.

Appendix A
Comfort

I said in the very beginning of this book that super sexual orgasm is a pleasure *every* woman can experience. And I know this to be true. Yet I also know that a small percentage of women will, after following the entire program in this book quite carefully, still struggle to experience the thrills of a true super sexual orgasm. While *any* woman can benefit from the exercises in this appendix, and I encourage all women to try them, this section has been included specifically for those women who need just a little more special help to fully realize their SSO goal.

I have written this book because I am a sex therapist. But I am also a woman who struggled to experience sexual pleasure. I think it is important for women reading this book to understand that I am *not* one of the lucky women I mentioned earlier who have always had natural access to the cul-de-sac and its extraordinary orgasmic potential. Nor is SSO something I was able to easily learn. I have had to work very hard to discover all of the pleasures I have written about in this book. But these pleasures have changed my relationships with men and, even more important, my relationship with myself.

All of my experience, both personal and professional, has taught me that the greatest stumbling block on the path to super sexual orgasm is *comfort*—comfort with your own body and its many gifts. And this is where we will end our journey to super sexual orgasm.

NO MORE MYSTERIES, NO MORE FEARS

The goal of this section is a simple one: I want to help you learn to accept, understand, and truly love your body. As I said before, there is more to SSO than learning to access the cul-de-sac. The more you love your body the more you will feel relaxed and at ease. And the more you feel relaxed and at ease, the easier it will be for you to achieve and embrace super sexual orgasm.

We are going to start at the surface and slowly work our way in to very intimate spaces. But I don't want you to just follow my instructions. I want you to understand *why* each exercise and technique has been included, and *why* each is so important.

One of the reasons super sexual orgasm has remained a secret for so long is because female sexual anatomy is an area that too many women shy away from. For some women, the territory is too sacred. For others, it is too scary. But every woman needs to fully understand how her body brings her pleasure and how it can bring her a lot more. And that means committing yourself to fully embracing your beautiful body and fully embracing your stunning sexuality.

LOOK WHO'S THERE

Are you alone right now? Are you in a private, safe place? Good. Then take off your clothes and let's get down to business with the following exercise.

I want you to stand in front of a mirror and observe your body. I don't mean glance. Really look. Bore holes in yourself from your concentration. Take your time—at least fifteen to twenty minutes. Study the arch of your shoulder and your pinkie nail on your left foot. Get out a hand mirror or even a magnifying glass if you wish. And as you observe, I want you to be nonjudgmental about what you see. That's really hard for many of us, I know. Whatever thoughts come into your mind, let them come, let them drift in and out: Just don't hang on to them. Don't get into a cycle of, "Aha! This thigh is why I'm never eating cookies again," or "My butt is definitely way too big." (We'll do an exercise soon where you can think all those thoughts, so don't think I'm cheating you of an opportunity to rag on yourself unmercifully like I know you do!) If you do have these feelings, just let them be right now. Don't focus on them. They are there and you are having them, but do not dwell on them. Instead, try your best to discover what an extraordinary gift the human body is. At the end of looking at your body inch by inch, close by taking a few minutes to look at your body as a whole. All that you have taken in about yourself is integrated in this last look.

What we are getting into here in this very first exercise is reevaluating the way you see yourself. No doubt like so many women and men you have negative attitudes about what you find in your reflection. Part of this we get from our particular upbringing and background. Much comes from the larger culture around us that places so much emphasis on a stylized and idealized female body the majority of women will never attain, though some might at great cost, financial and otherwise.

This exercise is a great healer when it comes to giving you a love for your body. Don't get me wrong. I am not saying that you cannot genuinely find aspects of your physical self that you want to change. There are a number of excellent books and other resources available on skin care, health, exercise, and clothing selection. You are an adult and you have a high degree of choice about how you look. While physical appearance is given way too much importance in our culture, making yourself look addition-ally attractive certainly can boost self-esteem and there is nothing wrong with that as long as you don't make it an obsession. To be very honest with you, I was once over-weight, flat-chested, had bad teeth—and my mother dressed me funny. When I got older, I made a decision to make some reasonable changes in my appearance and I've definitely felt better for it. But having made those changes I have reached a place of self-acceptance and personal comfort. Today, I do not look in the mirror and panic. When the fashion in models was Kate Moss, I did not say to myself "Barbara, you hippo!" Because Kate's body is fine for her and mine is fine for me. And I'm sure if you could really see who you are in the mirror, you would find that your body is actually terrific for you too.

For the next twenty minutes I want you to place your hands all over your body and let yourself feel the way your body feels. We're not doing any sensual stroking at this point. I just want you to make a comfortable touch connection with your body. Make sure you touch yourself everywhere. Your neck, your face, your stomach, your thighs, even the little spaces between your toes. Make a physical connection with every part of you, and hold that connection long enough to give yourself a clear memory of it. As you touch, let all thoughts come and go. There is no "goal" here, there is no "achievement level," there is no doing this "better" than anyone else. Relax and touch. Reintroduce the thinking you to the body you. Again, finish up by looking at your body as a whole. Admire the miracle that is you.

I hope that through the simple techniques in these exercises you can begin to develop the attitude that:

- your body looks and feels wonderfully good

- you can love your body the way it is

- you can have sensual and sexual enjoyment if you revel in who you are.

A client of mine, Betty, did not like to kiss and this caused problems for her in relationships. After doing the body image exercise you just completed, Betty revealed to me that she had been in a car accident as a teenager and had broken her nose. She had to have major reconstructive surgery. The surgeon had done an impeccable job and the scars of the trauma were no longer visible, but the trauma remained inside Betty's head. Betty felt that when her lovers were close enough to kiss her they could tell that her nose was reconstructed. Betty never told her lovers why she had such anxiety. The kissing issue always became a stumbling block in Betty's relationships and they all failed.

I am bringing this up because if this exercise reminds you of a traumatic experience or brings up powerful memories or emotions, you may find relief just in the expression of such feelings by getting them out in the open. If your anxieties remain great and unresolved, however, consider seeking the assistance of a qualified counselor or therapist so that you can deal with the issue completely. If such feelings are brought up by any of the exercises that follow in this book, *please go find the support you need.* There are many good people working in the therapeutic field who can ease your situation and work with you to release yourself from the tyranny of past traumas.

SPRING CLEANING

It's time to get a lot of good stuff and bad stuff out in the open. The day after you do the preceding exercises, I want you to complete this next exercise.

I want you to write out:

- everything you like and don't like about your body

- everything you like and don't like about your experience of sexuality and sensuality to this point in your life

- everything you want and don't want your experience of sexuality and sensuality to be in the future

Do this writing in a stream of consciousness. This is not Shakespeare you're creating, but rather a means of cleaning out your system. You're acknowledging where you're coming from so you can then set your sights on moving on. If you have a love affair with the shape of your left elbow, sing its praises on paper. If you have an eyebrow you arch just the smallest bit to make your lover come running, tell all about it. Write out your most embarrassing moments. And go ahead: be mean, rude, and darkly envious.

Get your feelings out, out, out! Let all your deeply held beliefs and secrets be told to yourself. Don't worry about complete sentences. Don't worry about spelling and punctuation. Write furiously, with focus and honesty.

If you are more of a visual than a word person, take a stack of magazines including fashion-glamour, culinary-travel, and nature, go through them and image associate for each of the three categories outlined above. Circle the pictures or parts of pictures that speak to you as you see them, then go back and cut them out and glue them into a collage, perhaps even embellishing with your own drawing and captioning. You could do your collage in terms of the colors that the categories bring up for you— or perhaps you'll respond by circling shapes and textures. Do this exercise with as much wild and creative abandon as you want as long as it connects with your feelings. As with the writing, though, don't dwell on the pictures.

You're going for a first instinct connection here. You see it and know it means something to you, so circle it!

If you are more of a verbal person, do a spoken-word stream of consciousness. Tape record it so that you can play it back afterward and hear what you've said. The reason I suggest this is some of my clients have gotten into an almost trancelike state using this verbal approach and then afterward don't really remember what they've said.

If you want to do the writing, the collage, *and* the spoken-word exercise, good for you. You're really getting to the heart of what you feel, the better to implement great changes in your life.

GETTING TO KNOW YOU

Let me state again here that it is so very important, when your goal is achieving super sexual orgasm, to spend time reintroducing yourself on a very intimate level to your own physical self. For the more connected you are to your body, the more adept you will be at accessing your SSO capabilities. Women who achieve SSO most easily, regularly, and intensely are women who have a harmonious relationship with their bodies. It's not a coincidence, it's part of the SSO process.

Let's do a test. When was the last time you were turned on by your own skin? Take that a step further. When was the last time you could get turned on by your own skin by just thinking about it? You see, women who are at ease with their own sexuality are not necessarily the most gorgeous women in the world. I'm sure at one or another moment in your life you have seen or met one of these women. Some are actually quite average looking but they exude such charm, such enveloping sensuality, that their presence draws you in and makes you want to be around them. These women can turn others on because they are excited to be in their own bodies. And this comes from knowing their bodies. They love each curve and valley. Even their moles! They love their skin, their toes, their thighs. They know the feel of themselves from head to toe.

You've heard the expression that from knowledge comes power. That is certainly true in the sexual arena. And nobody can give you that "drawing power" like you can. It's this simple. When you know your body, when you love your body, you and your body become something other people want to love. You've heard some of your women friends say, and perhaps you have said yourself, that they feel more attractive when they are wearing this or that piece of clothing or jewelry. It accents the line of a neck or slims hips or brings out the aqua in the eyes. There is no magic going on. That necklace is not talismanic. You are giving that bauble your permission to put you at ease, to make you think in your own mind that you look fabulous. And when you think you are fabulous, you *are* fabulous. And people will find you so.

Love, acceptance, and permission. These are three words that should guide you always. The journey to SSO is a very personal undertaking, perhaps one of the most intimate experiences you will have. Would you go on such a journey with a stranger? No. And yet, no matter what you think you know about yourself as you read this, I guarantee you that you are in some measure distanced from your true self and body self. So let me give you a wild sentence that might seem out of *Through the Looking Glass:* You are going to go through some unbecoming in order to become. Which is to say, you are going to reestablish a level of ease, understanding, and trust with yourself in order to allow you to achieve the depth of self-intimacy SSO requires. You are going to get to know yourself inside and out.

The exercises you have just completed, and the exercises that follow shortly, will enable you to give yourself permission to feel as sexy and as beautiful as you are. Because once you realize what a sexual knockout you are, whether dressed to the nines or in sweats with your legs spiny as a porcupine and your hair looking like you've been coifed in the Sahara, you are going to have that natural level of self-confidence and centeredness upon which you can start to build up to your spectacular SSO.

SIZING UP THE SITUATION

A note on fitness before we go on. You don't have to be a marathoner to have a wild SSO ride. I myself am the most casual of exercisers, taking just a few hour-long walks along the beach every week. But I am generally able to maintain my weight in proportion to my height and physique. What I am getting at is the closer you are to a sensible body size and good physical tone, the easier you will find doing the SSO exercises in this book, the more dynamic the experience will be, and the more pleasurable your sex life as a whole will become.

Now lovemaking itself is a great workout because of all the movement involved. Frequent and vigorous sessions exercise the long muscles of your arms and legs, giving your body a more sculpted look. Making love steps up your metabolism and can even help ward off osteoporosis. It's a terrific physical toner because of the connection to your respiration and blood flow. Sex deepens your breathing and increases the oxygen you take in, oxygen that then flows throughout your body. Your hair is shinier, your eyes are brighter, and your skin is radiant because of your increased circulation. The sensation of arousal you experience from sex results from the release of endorphins from your brain. Endorphins can make you experience altered states of consciousness such as "runner's high" as well as boost your immune system and act as natural painkillers.

But even with all the physiological benefits of sex, in addition to being the ultimate, intimate thrill, don't rely on lovemaking to be your sole exercise workout. No matter the physical shape you're in, increase your exercise time by saying "I'm going to do ten more minutes of some kind of workout three times a week from this moment on." That's only half an hour a week! No big deal. So do it.

Of course, as wonderful as exercise is, there are some things it cannot do for your health. It can't make up for eating junk food, smoking, doing drugs, or using alcohol excessively. And the best sex can't make up for these negative health practices either. Use the empowered feelings you will increasingly have as you move through the SSO exercises to inspire you to shed any remaining bad health habits and implement beneficial ones in their place.

R-E-S-P-E-C-T

Now please, do not interpret my words about exercise and body shape and tone as another demand on you to be and look perfect. No, I just want you to be healthy and physically comfortable to the degree that it works for you, a very individual thing. We women get "be perfect" directives constantly on subtle and not-so-subtle levels from our society. We're more liberated than we were fifty years ago on many levels, but we still have a long way to go when it comes to personal acceptance and self-respect. Most women I talk to in my practice and lectures have a problem with their body image. Even some of the most stunning women I meet find something to dislike about themselves. I remember one woman whose body I would have traded my soul for telling me with great sadness in her voice "I don't feel okay about having sex because I don't feel comfortable about having my partner look at my body."

Don't allow negative body perceptions to stand in the way of achieving your SSO. Don't deny yourself the permission to enjoy your complete sexuality because you think you haven't achieved society's standard of attractiveness. Your sexuality is a terrible thing to waste. The sensate focus exercises we are going to do next will allow you to transform your relationship with your body and your connection to it. Get ready to take your first step toward making yourself truly whole. And remember, as you engage in these exercises, be gentle and generous with yourself.

REACH OUT AND TOUCH YOURSELF . . . AGAIN

What I would like to do with you now is take some time to revisit the techniques of sensate focus, and explore their magic in greater depth. Give yourself at least one full hour for this next exercise.

Sit or lie naked in a comfortable position. Place your fingertips on your body gently and focus in on that point of contact. Follow the point of contact wherever it moves. If your mind wanders off, gently bring your focus back to what you are physically feeling at the contact point.

Keep your touch slow. Slow, slow, slow. Being touched in this manner is comforting and relaxing, which is necessary if you are to reach profound levels of arousal and SSO. Don't massage, but rather keep to a light, constant motion. You can use long sweeping strokes or short ones (try both styles to see what they do for you). Remember to breathe evenly.

Try closing your eyes and cutting your pace—even if you think it is super-slow already—in half. As you touch, let your sensory awareness include temperature, texture, shape, movement. The only intention about this kind of touching is that you are touch-ing to make yourself feel good. Remember to maintain contact with some part of your body the entire time.

Sensate focus touching can be done on any part of your body with any part of your body. You can touch with your fingertips, your hand, your face, your hair, your nose, whatever you want. Do not avoid parts of your body when you are doing the exercise. Touch whatever you want in whatever order but make sure you touch yourself everywhere.

When you get to your genital area, remember this is not an occasion for masturbation. You will just caress slowly and let yourself appreciate the touch. Be especially careful to have clean hands and add a touch of baby oil or other lubricant before you proceed. Slowly begin to touch your inner thighs and your vaginal lips. Keep your focus on what you are touching. Relax. Breathe. Slowly stroke your clitoris and inner lips. Insert a finger into your vagina and let it move in and out. Spend lots of time going over your genital terrain. If you become aroused, that's fine, but this is not the goal. Your only goal is to experience and appreciate the sensations.

Whatever occurs during this sensate focus exercise is all part of getting in touch with your pleasure, enjoying yourself, and learning about your body. As you explore your genital area in general and your vagina in particular you'll be struck by the smell of this area. The odor of a clean, healthy vagina may be strong, but it is very posi-tive. Save your money and don't use sprays or deodor-ants. Keeping your genital area washed and, if you desire, shaved, is all you need to do.

You may still feel awkward touching yourself. In my practice, I see many women who have never touched their genitals without feeling embarrassed, "dirty," or guilty. I can also say from my clinical experiences that few women explore their bodies as a whole enough to discover what turns them on. This lack of self-knowledge is often the only thing stopping them from becoming aroused enough to reach orgasmic Shangri-La.

If you can't do a prolonged self-touching stretch, start with ten minutes. Do it for a few days and then go for fifteen minutes. Little by little, work your way up to a half hour. You will be surprised and delighted at what you gain when you do. Sensate focus self-touching will help you learn more about your body, become more comfortable with it, and realize its allure and sheer wonderfulness.

You may, through these exercises, discover the whole other country of touching that is a source of relaxation and of physical and mental well-being. Your comfort level with desiring and being desired will also increase. Self-touching will also ease any subtle, subsurface anxieties and apprehensions that may have kept you from touching other people in a friendly, nonsexual setting.

As I mentioned to you earlier in the book, stop immediately if you become very agitated or unduly anxious. A little nervousness or unease is okay to work through, but something more means there may indeed be something more going on. If you don't settle down after a short while, do consider contacting a therapist to discuss what may be happening and what you can do to address the situation.

ZEN AND THE ART OF SENSATE FOCUS

Anxiety-free touching liberates. A person or persons can revel in an experience of tenderness, caring, and gentleness without interference from concerns about performance or adequacy. When you are touching yourself, similarly unburden yourself of expectations about what you should be or want to be or thought you might be feeling and *just feel*.

At all times stay in the here and now. This goes for self-touching and for touching with a partner. Concentrate on the part of the body you are touching at the moment, not the area you finished touching or the area coming up. If you start having thoughts like "I'm nervous about touching my own breasts," or "My hips are so fat," you are removing yourself from the sensate focus and getting into your head, causing distancing in the first case and being judgmental in the second. Consciously bring your attention back to the point of contact between your fingers and your body. Don't get upset at yourself if your mind drifts. Just bring it back. Everybody gets distracted, even longtime practitioners of sensate focus. Your ability to bring yourself back and then to stay in touch with the moment, however, will certainly improve with practice.

Staying in the here and now also means that you are focusing on the touching encounter you are having right now, not the one you have had in the past or future. *Fully experiencing your sexuality as it happens to you is the key to pleasure.*

As you totally inhabit your body, you can entirely experience the exquisite sensations of being touched in a loving way. This in itself may be a novel experience for many women, including yourself. I told you the journey to SSO would change your life in many ways! After completing sensate focus exercises, most women experience a heightened awareness. Many feel better about themselves immediately. Others have expressed to me that they feel a kindness toward themselves they never felt before. I've worked with clients for whom this caressing, especially in the genital area, prompts tearfulness and sadness. This is part of the healing process, essential to self-integration.

LETTING GO

To experience deep pleasure, you must be deeply relaxed. It doesn't matter how well you learn the exercises in this book. If you are keyed up, overwrought, or anxious when you make love, utilizing the exercises won't get the SSO you have inside of you. Sure, you'll eke out something, but only a fraction of what you really have to offer yourself.

If it has been a long time since you've felt really relaxed, let me remind you what it feels like. You breathe deeply, your muscles relax, and your heart slows to a gentler pace. You may find you have few thoughts at all or that they just drift by randomly without taking hold.

You can take yourself to a place of deep relaxation through the sensate focus touching exercises you just experienced. I have seen with my therapeutic clients time and again how making these touching experiences a part of lovemaking sends both partners to a place of relaxation, which in turn increases their enjoyment of all that follows. The understanding by both partners that sensate focus touching is not some mandatory foreplay to do in order to get the "real stuff" is key. For these sexually fulfilled couples, sensate focus touching is an integral, eagerly anticipated, and enjoyed experience in and of itself.

To successfully complete the exercises in this book, you need to come from a relaxed state of being. You are reading this book *for* your enjoyment and to *heighten* your enjoyment. You are in the realm of experiencing as opposed to mastering. No one is going to the head of the class here. You have your own seat, and you'll finish in your own seat. All I hope is that it becomes an increasingly pleasurable seat for you. That is my only expectation and it should be your only expectation as well.

EVERY BREATH YOU TAKE

Good breathing technique and relaxation go hand in hand. To say that breath is the essence of life is seemingly to say the obvious. But if that is so, I must tell you most of the people I meet in my work really need a refresher course on the obvious. They come into my office taking short or shallow breaths or breathing erratically. It's no wonder that they are encountering sexual difficulties! Proper breathing is the basis of life—and of feeling alive. So it stands to reason that when we are choked up, tense, or choppy in our breathing, our sex life is choked up, tense, and choppy. Try getting aroused when you can barely take in a decent breath of air!

Earlier in this book you learned belly breathing. Right now, I want you to learn caress breathing. Belly breathing and caress breathing have a myriad of uses. Don't just save them for SSO, make them a part of your daily life. They will release the benevolent natural energies in your body. Both techniques help you take more oxygen into your body. In addition to an enhanced sexual response, you will also find that these breathing techniques will lower your heart rate and blood pressure. You may like one more than the other or you may like them both. You decide.

For this exercise, be sure to choose a quiet location with minimal distractions. Wear loose-fitting clothing. Take your phone off the hook or turn the ringer down.

Begin with a few minutes of belly breathing. Now try this: Blow all the air out of your lungs through your nose rapidly. Now slowly take all the air you can back in through your nose. Imagine you are caressing the inside of your lungs with air. Remember to relax your stomach muscles. As soon as the air has filled your lungs, start breathing out again slowly. Don't hold your breath. Do this caress breathing five or six times in succession. You can almost feel your heart rate decrease and your blood pressure fall. This breathing technique is so simple and yet is a powerful means of regulating the rhythms and responses of your body.

DON'T MUSCLE IN ON YOURSELF

You can be relaxed, you can be breathing easily, and yet if some of your muscles are tensed up, you will still be doing yourself in. How can that be, you ask? Surely if your muscles were tense you would notice. You would notice if this tensing of muscles was something out of the ordinary. But, unfortunately, many of us have become acclimated to this unnatural body state. We only notice how uncomfortable and restrictive it is when we take action to release the muscles.

We spoke earlier in this section about how the healthy energy, body stamina, and physical tone that come from fitness increase your pleasure during lovemaking. Deeply relaxed muscles also heighten the amorous capacity of a sexual encounter. As you become aware of how your muscles feel when they are not tense, you will consciously be able to relax them when necessary so muscle tension will not interfere with your life in general and lovemaking in particular.

Lie down on your back in a comfortable position on your bed. Starting with the muscles in your right foot, tighten these muscles as much as you can for a few seconds and then release them, the entire time maintaining a pattern of easy, calm breathing. Go to your left foot and repeat the tensing and releasing. In this manner, work your way up your entire body, inch by inch, muscle by muscle. Slowly explore your calves, thighs, entire legs, buttocks, abdomen, stomach, chest, hands, lower and upper arms, shoulders, neck, and face. You'll probably find some muscles you never knew about—and never realized held so much tension.

While it is ideal to lie on your bed to do the exercise, and I would suggest that you learn to do it this way, once you are familiar with your body's musculature you can do this tension releaser any time, any place. It is extremely helpful to relax the body before working on your SSO techniques, but the uses and benefits of this exercise are endless. Think of it as your quickie spa vacation. Restful and rejuvenating. And you did it all yourself.

THE GIFT THAT KEEPS ON GIVING

This concludes the exercises for body comfort. Over time, you will integrate their benefits into all aspects of your lovemaking. This integration will yield magic in many places, and also bring you to the SSO experience you seek.

Your body is the finest present you have. Very few people are fully aware of its luxurious bounty, its selfless giving, its daily full support. Move from the ranks of those who don't value their body fully to those who appreciate its gifts. Your body craves recognition and attention to its capacity for touch, closeness, connection, sexuality, and sensuality. And when you give back to yourself, you will find you have so much more to share with others in your life as well.

In the course of this section, I hope you have also begun to see how deriving joy and pleasure from a sexual experience means you must trust and value yourself—your body and your feelings. Sex is not about self-sacrifice. Sex is not about placing greater emphasis on another's pleasure. Sex is about two human beings experiencing pleasure in equal measure, on equal ground.

And SSO is only as fulfilling as the context in which you experience it. The best are experienced in an atmosphere of kindness, love, and caring.

Dedicate yourself to finding such a place in your life.

Appendix B
Toys

The following is a list of popular companies that sell dildos, vibrators, and other sex toys through the mail. While I do not feel comfortable personally endorsing any of these companies, I have conducted trouble-free business with all of them. Call or write for catalogues.

Good Vibrations
San Francisco, CA
1–415–974–8990
(call for catalogue)

Intimate Treasures
San Francisco, CA
1–415–863–5002
(call for catalogue)

Xandria Collection
Department C 1096
P.O. Box 31039
San Francisco, CA 94131–9988
(write for catalogue)

Lady Calston
908 Niagara Falls Blvd., Suite 519
North Tonawanda, NY 14120–2060
1–800–690–5239

Adam and Eve
P.O. Box 900
Department CS 357
Carrboro, NC 27510
1–800–274–0333